JUICE YOUR WAY
THROUGH

Pregnancy and Beyond

Includes baby friendly RAW JUICES & SMOOTHIES

Zoë Clarke

Published by ROC Publishing 2016

Acknowledgments

Thank you to my clients for your ideas, inspiration and energy. Especially Annabel – it's taken me a while...

Thanks Teflon Don and Aisha Kan't

Good luck and congratulations Vicky – I hope this book comes in useful....

Table of Contents

Acknowledgments 4

Table of Contents 7

Foreword 19

Chapter 1 - An Introduction to Juicing............................21

What exactly is Juicing?...22

What Does Juicing Involve? 22

So, What Can You Juice?..23

How Healthy is Juicing? 23

The Juicing Craze 25

Why Juice During Pregnancy? 25

Is it Safe?...27

The One "Catch" to Juicing During Pregnancy 27

Chapter 2 - Responsible Juicing..................................29

The Pregnancy Juicing "Do" List.............................29

Use Organic Produce 30

Make Juicing a Regular Part of Your Diet....................30

Use Juice to Fill Nutritional Gaps................................30

Use Herbs 31

Control Your Sugar Intake 31

The Pregnancy Juicing "Don't" List 31

Don't do a Prolonged Juice Fast.................................31

Don't Drink Store Bought Juices 32

Don't Use Turmeric in Juices 32

Drink Your Juices as Soon as Possible......................32

Choosing the Best Juicer 33

The Three Types of Juicers 34

The Importance of Organic Juices............................35

Worried About the Taste?...37

Chapter 3 - Selection Time..39

Fruits for Juicing 39

Avocados 40

Babies Delight: Creamy Avocado and Banana
Smoothie...41

Mangoes 41

MORNING MANGO – ANTI-SICKENESS 42

Grapes...42

Lime...43

LIMES FOR EINSTIENS..44

Bananas...44

Oranges...44

Apple...45

Vegetables for Juicing 45

Celery 45

Carrot 46

Cucumber 47

Recipes 48

COOL AS A CARROT 48

THE GREEN SPIRITED BABY 49

THE ACID SOOTHER 49

Fruits and Vegetables to avoid when pregnant 49

Pineapples 50

Papaya 50

RAW Vegetables 50

Herbs for Juicing 51

Ginger 51

MORNING GINGER ZINGER 52

HOMEMADE GINGER ALE 53

Yam/ Sweet potato 53

YUMMY MUMMY YAM-YAM JUICE 54

Red Raspberry 54

RASBERRY NIPPLE 55

A Few Things to Remember 55

Chapter 4 - Make the Most of Juicing 57

Common Juicing Mistakes 57

Adding Excessive Amounts of Sugar 58

Table of Contents

Gulping Down Your Juice 58

Buying Pasteurized and Preserved Juices 59

Preparation Advice 59

Tips for Storing Juice 60

Buying Quality Produce 61

Quality of Utensils 62

"Extras" to take Your Juice up a Level 62

Cacao 62

Goji-Berries 64

Maca 64

Chia 64

GOOD MORNING MACA 65

GOGI, MACA and CACOA SMOOTHIE 65

SUPER GREEN SMOOTHIE 66

AVOCADO & MACA SMOOTHIE 66

Prenatal Vitamin Juices 66

GINGER PEACH PASSION 67

BANANA & APRICOT FREEZE 68

GRAPEFRUIT, CARROTT & GINGER JUICE 68

Juicing and Pregnancy FAQs 68

Chapter 5 - Pregnancy and Nutrition 71

Folic Acid 71

Magnesium 71

Zinc 72

Vitamin B12 72

Omega 3 72

BABY BEET JUICE 73

CUCUMBER REFRESHER 73

HOT GINGER ZINGER 74

Chapter 6 - Dealing with Pregnancy Related Issues 75

Combating Fatigue 75

CAULIFLOWER & BROCCOLI JUICE 76

POPEYE PICKER-UPPER 76

BANANA BLISS SMOOTHIE 77

Morning Sickness 77

SUPER CELERY JUICE 78

FEELING FENNEL FANTASTIC 78

High Blood Pressure and Pre-Eclampsia 79

NO PRESSURE COCKTAIL 80

POWER ME UP JUICE 80

CALMER KALE JUICE 81

WATER BABY SMOOTHIE 83

Iron Deficiency 83

THE SPICY IRON 84

Table of Contents

Constipation 85

    BOWEL DOWN 86

SMOOTH OPERATOR 86

PEAR, SPINACH & PRUNE JUICE 87

CITRUS CUCUMBER COOLER 87

Blood Circulation 88

    THE CITRUS CIRCULATOR 89

    GINGER PARADISE 89

    FULL IMMUNITY ENERGIZER.....................90

Non-Specific Dermatitis 90

    SHINY SKIN JUICE 91

RAINBOW BLITZ 92

Breast Milk Issues 92

    Mastitis 92

    Low Supply of Milk 93

Too Much Milk 93

Clogged Ducts 93

    THE BETTER BREAST 94

The Pregnancy Mask (Chloasma) 94

    MAGIC MASK MIX 95

    Depression and Anxiety 95

Fertility 96

Hereditary...96

Relationship Blues...96

Past Miscarriages 97

Specific Pregnancy Problems 97

Symptoms of Stress and Depression 97

    KARMA GREEN 98

    SLEEPY TIME JUICE 98

    Headaches 98

    CARROT HEAD SMOOTHIE 100

    THE HYDRATOR 100

Insomnia 100

Morning Sickness (at Night…)..............................101

Excessive Urination.......................................101

Restless Leg Syndrome 101

Natural Insomnia Cures 101

Cramping 102

    CELERY CRAMPER 102

Urinary Tract Infections 103

    CRANBERRY RELIVER 103

Indigestion and Heartburn 103

    ALOE ACID 104

Overheating 106

SCRUB 'N' SHINE SMOOTHIE..................................106

SWISS SKIN 107

Chapter 7 - Post-Pregnancy Juicing 109

Managing Your Dietary Intake.............................109

Breastfeeding and Juicing..................................111

BERRY BLASTER SMOOTHIE 112

Chapter 8 - Juicing Vegetables for Babies 113

Key Nutrients...114

Calcium 114

Zinc..115

Vitamins A, D, E and K 115

Iron 116

Vitamin B & C 116

Considerations and Recommendations.................116

Quantity...116

Sweetness..117

Concentration 117

Packaged or Fresh 117

Strain the Juices 117

Use One Vegetable at a Time............................118

Baby Friendly Recipes..118

BABY CARROT JUICE..118

LITTLE GREEN MACHINE 118

ABC JUICE 119

GRACIOUS GRAPES 119

Chapter 9: Dealing With Post-Pregnancy Issues 121

Post-Baby Weight Loss 121

GO TO JUICE...122

THE PARSLEY SOOTHER 122

Water Retention 122

THE GRATEFUL GRAPEFUL 123

THE EXTINGUISHER 123

GINGER PLUS...124

Stretch Marks...124

THE ELASTIC TOMATO SMOOTHIE......................125

HONEYDEW HEAVEN SMOOTHIE.......................125

RED RAW SMOOTHIE 125

Dry Skin 126

HYDRATING GREEN JUICE..................................126

CUCUMBER MEDLEY..126

CARROT & CELERY STICK JUICE 127

VITAMIN SKIN JUICE..127

Fatigue 127

KIWI ENERGIZER SMOOTHIE 128

BERRY BERRY TIRED SMOOTHIE 128

CITRUS & KALE JUICE 128

Insomnia 129

CHERRY BOMBASTIC SMOOTHIE...........................129

CHERRY BLASTER 129

SPROUTED CAULIFLOWER JUICE 129

Urinary Incontinence...130

BROCCOLI ON THE ROCKS 131

ASPIRATIONAL ASPARAGUS 131

GINGER PARADISE 131

Afterword 133

Glossary...135

Index..152

Foreword

Juicing is a PASSION

I started RAW vegetable juicing soon after I was diagnosed with Adenoid Cystic Carcinoma – a relatively rare and relentless type of cancer that likes to run its course. This shocking news prompted me to explore every single avenue of opportunity in supporting my body to heal…and lucky for me, I found RAW juicing alongside a healthy plant based diet. I also adore RAW super nutritious smoothies….

It felt natural for me to look towards food as potential medicine, particularly by choosing natural plant based food. My body felt totally toxic – I needed to clean it and to provide it with living nutrients and vitamins if I was going to recover. For me, RAW juicing was the key. Overall, it helped me to turn a particularly overwhelming and negative time into a hugely positive and life changing experience.

I am now a Qualified Natural Juice Therapist registered with the Complementary Medical Association. I offer consultations on a whole range of conditions. I love to spread the word.

I juice almost every day and when I don't juice I really miss it. I also enjoy creating nutritious and delicious recipes and juices for followers of my online blog

WWW.HOTDAYCOLDDAY.COM

Also on all social media sites as
HOT DAY COLD DAY

Pregnancy and juicing is a topic that comes up frequently - *"Is it safe to Juice if I am pregnant?"* – I've had loads of emails about this.

The answer is a big and definite, infinite **YES**

Juicing will benefit you **both** tremendously and I couldn't encourage you enough to consider RAW juicing. The fact you are reading this is an exciting step on the path to nutritional health. It seriously has no boundaries.

You will not only improve your own health, but that of your baby. Juicing and consuming nutritious healthy smoothies whilst pregnant requires a little more mindfulness and consideration regarding the different nutritional needs at different stages – each trimester will have different challenges for you both. It may sound hard at first, but I promise it'll soon become second nature – it'll feel as easy as popping on the kettle.

This book will hopefully support you in your juicing journey. Both in preparing for your pregnancy, during pregnancy and in supporting your body to heal once you have given birth.

I wish you both a healthy pregnancy and exciting adventures ahead - both in LIFE and in JUICING
Zoë Clarke
Natural Juice Therapist

Chapter 1 - An Introduction to Juicing

The hype about juicing has taken the health world by an absolute storm. It's not only limited to health-conscious individuals anymore. The average person is now curious about juicing and how to make super healthy juices, curious as to what makes it a preferred health habit for so many people. I see the benefits of juicing first hand - both personally and professionally. So let's briefly look at what this popular practice entails.

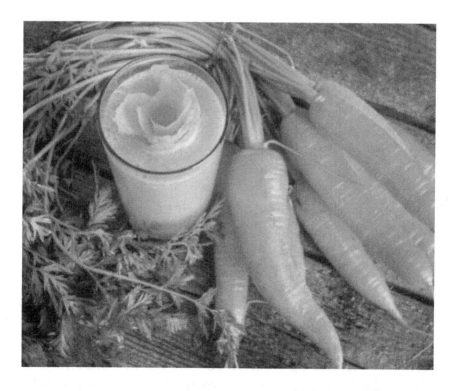

What exactly is Juicing?

In simple terms, juicing is the extraction of juice from the tissue of RAW fruits and vegetables with a juicer. The pure liquid contains nutrients in dense concentration that are easy to consume and digest. These include antioxidants, vitamins, minerals, phytonutrients and anti-inflammatory compounds.

Juicing is quick - it's loaded with health benefits and best of all it's incredibly simple to incorporate into your daily routine.

What Does Juicing Involve?

Juicing is usually done with a juicing machine, although some people prefer to hand juice. Personally I like both. It just depends on how much time I have and where I am. I also love to blend some vegetables with fruit and super foods, I use a VITAMIX which delivers a delicious smoothie every time - packed with plant power and natural protein, BUT more about that later.

The most time consuming steps when juicing are preparing and washing the produce - also cleaning the equipment after use. But I've got to be honest, I've never really found this a huge problem, I can easily make a fresh vegetable juice and clean up in just 10 minutes on the way to work. The same time it'd take to make a fresh coffee and toast a Bagel.

My first essential tip is ALWAYS attempt to consume the juice when it is fresh for the greatest flavour and health benefits.

So, What Can You Juice?

This is the exciting bit.

You can juice ALMOST ANY fruit or vegetable you can imagine.

WOW, that's good news hey? Just imagine the endless variety and constant new combinations that you can concoct. Leftover fruit and vegetables? NO problem when you have a juicer and a blender to hand. Using your creativity and ingenuity to come up with new recipes keeps you seriously interested and on track.

Begin with easy recipes you find online (or even better in this book) and from there, just try to have fun. Experiment. Honestly, it gets easier. Popular combinations include leafy greens like spinach with cucumber, carrot, or apple for sweetness. After you've read this book you'll be less anxious about what exactly you can and can't eat for the health of your baby (and of course your own future health).

How Healthy is Juicing?

Juiced RAW fruits and vegetables are **far** superior to vitamin and mineral supplements in any form. The earth is providing you with an abundance of natural, non toxic health treats in non-tablet form – what more could you wish for? RAW juice is amazingly easy for your body to digest and absorb – providing a punchy and powerful boost to the immune system.

Juicing is much healthier than eating or cooking the

same foods. Research at Minnesota State University found drinking fresh juices allows for 90% nutrient absorption. **Eating the same foods returns a rate of only 35% - that's an incredible difference of 55% - WOW.**

The National Institute of Health studied daily recommended essential nutrients. Most people get less than 75% of the total amount suggested. Juicing makes it so much easier to reach the recommended five daily servings of fruits and vegetables. Although to be honest if you're a regular juicer you really won't need to worry about this. Moreover, cooking produce destroys much of the original nutrients content – the more RAW produce you can consume the better. But that's another book altogether.

Juices are fibre-free and self-digesting. Fruits and vegetables offer enzymes that aid in carbohydrate, fat, and protein digestion. This creates greater protection against ulcers, acid reflux disease and gallstones.

Juicing will enhance your immune system functioning which in turn helps to fight infectious diseases. Detoxifying juices cleanse the organs, while the liquid keeps them hydrated. Fresh juices increase energy and stamina, normalize sleep patterns and enhance both learning and memory.

Do you really need any more reasons to juice?

The Juicing Craze

The rising popularity of juicing raises many questions. Is it a fad or a craze? Does it carry real nutritional benefits? The answers, in orders, are "no" and "YES."

Juicing is no longer a special interest nutritional practice. The health benefits have made this a mainstream dietary choice that delivers proven benefits.

- **Better energy and stamina**
- **Improved skin tone and health**
- **Enhanced immunity**
- **Stronger digestion**

And, of course, juicing supports **HEALTHY WEIGHT LOSS.** I'm happy to say it's well and truly here to stay.

Organic RAW juicing can only have BENEFITS and does NO harm at all.

Why Juice During Pregnancy?

During pregnancy, it really is critical to try and take care of your health as much as practicably possible – a healthy Mum will hopefully equal a healthy baby. Although please remember it's also important not to put too much pressure on yourself either. There are many methods to ensure your good health and proper nourishment during pregnancy. Incorporating RAW juices and nutritious smoothies will only help and it won't deprive your growing child of crucial nutrients.

Vitamin C pretty much tops the list of nutrients for pregnant women in supporting your immune system and protecting your baby.

Vitamin A comes in a close second. Fruits and vegetables are an excellent source of folic acid. Folic acid helps the placenta to carry nutrients from the mother's body to the unborn child.

Juicing spinach, broccoli, beets, oranges and strawberries guarantees exceptional folic acid levels.

Iron protects your baby from anemia and enhances the production of oxygen-rich hemoglobin. Iron also helps to prevent pre-term labour.

Juicing spinach, beans, peas and leeks creates a powerful Iron cocktail.

Pregnant women are notorious for craving unusual foods; unfortunately, these choices are rarely healthy. The great news is that some juices can, by design, **stop cravings**. The pantothenic acid and Vitamin B5 in broccoli, avocados or lentils fulfills salt cravings.

Apples, grapes, broccoli, potatoes and green beans help to lessen the desire for sugar.

Juicing truly can play a critical role in keeping you and your baby healthy and nourished. Helping you to stay fit and strong and potentially avoiding health problems before they develop.

Is it Safe?

All expectant mothers have serious questions about dietary or lifestyle changes. That's a good thing! The reason you're reading this book is to help educate yourself and make an informed decision. In the following pages you'll learn that juicing is not only safe, but also extremely healthy (and great fun too...)

During pregnancy your daily nutritional will rise considerably. A growing fetus has considerable developmental needs that juicing can help you both meet in a safe and very tasty manner. I recommend juices from **organic fruits and vegetables** to provide a spectrum of nutrients and minerals. Consumed fresh, they offer maximal support for you and your child.

The One "Catch" to Juicing During Pregnancy

Never ever, embark on a juice fast during pregnancy.

The key is to incorporate juicing into your daily diet. Follow a healthy food regime that includes juices as well as eating RAW fruits and vegetables. Aim to increase your knowledge about your nutritional needs during pregnancy and focus on the fruits and vegetables that will meet these.

Don't drink juices as a meal replacement strategy during pregnancy. This will only put further strain on your body.
The keys to safe juicing during pregnancy are:

- **Balancing your nutritional needs**
- **Using organic and high quality produce - if you**

are unable to do this make sure you wash the vegetables and fruit well

- **Maintaining immaculate juicing equipment**

Combined with a healthy eating plan, juicing will become an important supporting strategy for a healthy pregnancy – **and beyond.**

Chapter 2 - Responsible Juicing

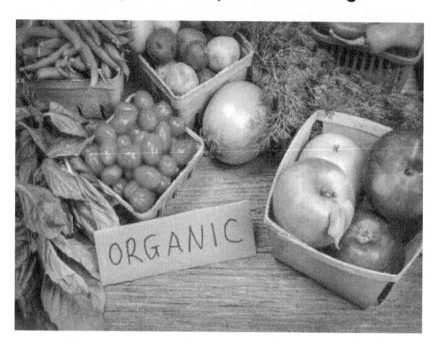

It's important to approach juicing in a responsible way; however, making sensible well-informed choices as well as managing the rest of your busy life can be a challenge. It's important to try and make it as easy as possible, you want juicing to be fun and sustainable – not a chore to dread. Pregnancy is hard enough without any additional anxieties. With that in mind, let's review some important "do" and "don't" rules.

The Pregnancy Juicing "Do" List

What you choose to put into your body during this sensitive period affects both you and your unborn baby. Never lose sight of this, when you're reaping the benefits of a fresh, RAW juice bursting with live enzymes you'll **both** be glowing inside and out.

Use Organic Produce

Selecting organic fruits and vegetables minimizes exposure to toxins. Eliminating these substances from your diet is a sound health practice under normal circumstances. During pregnancy, it's even more important. Studies have shown that when exposed to toxic foods in utero, a child's cognitive capacity can suffer.

If you are unable to get hold of organic produce, then don't worry – just take the time to wash each vegetable well before juicing – this will significantly reduce the chemical load.

Make Juicing a Regular Part of Your Diet

When you make the decision to incorporate juicing in your diet, commit to drinking fresh RAW juice on a regular basis. This will ensure that your body receives tip top levels of nutrients in a truly optimal form. Juices deliver vitamin and mineral content without loading you down with unnecessary calories. When it comes to RAW juicing I really don't believe there is any need to count calories.

Use Juice to Fill Nutritional Gaps

Use juicing at least twice a day between regular meals. This prevents hunger and you will be less likely to binge on unhealthy foods. It also creates the opportunity to take in superior levels of essential nutrients like Vitamin A, Vitamin C, and folic acid.

Use Herbs

Herbs, especially ginger can be a great addition to your juicing process. Ginger relieves nausea and prevents vomiting. Early in your pregnancy, it will help with morning sickness during pregnancy. Ginger also soothes the intestines and helps in eliminating gas from the body.
Ginger is a true wonder.

Control Your Sugar Intake

Control your sugar intake to prevent gestational diabetes. To avoid high sugar content in your juices, use roughly a ratio of **80% vegetable to 20% fruit.**

The Pregnancy Juicing "Don't" List

In this list of juicing "best practices" during pregnancy, there are also several things to avoid, so pay particular attention to the following points.

Don't do a Prolonged Juice Fast

A prolonged juice fast releases toxins into the bloodstream. Fasting during pregnancy could potentially put your child at risk as the blood supply to the fetus can become polluted with these toxins. The fasting also puts your body under considerable stress at a time when you really need to be supporting it as much as possible. I'm sure there are people that have done this safely, however for me I feel It's better to play safe; personally I wouldn't recommend using juicing as an alternative to food whilst pregnant.

Don't Drink Store Bought Juices

I always try to avoid store bought juices, simply because you don't know their source. Unpasteurized fresh juices may contain harmful bacteria. Whilst pregnant I advise clients to only drink juices you prepare yourself. This is the only way you can be certain about the quality of the produce and the cleanliness of the equipment.

Don't Use Turmeric in Juices

Turmeric contains a major active component called curcumin. Using Turmeric in your everyday recipes or externally isn't an issue – it's safe. However, I wouldn't advice JUICING fresh turmeric - this would deliver a particularly concentrated dose which in turn could possibly cause uterine contractions. However, on a positive note turmeric creates lovely soft, supple skin. Try mixing a paste of turmeric and coconut cream – this can be gently massaged into your stomach as a preventive for stretch marks.

Drink Your Juices as Soon as Possible

The process of oxidation occurs the very moment you begin to juice, therefore try and drink your juice as soon after extraction as possible - if you're anything like me you'll be drinking it at the same time as juicing – I just can't resist. If you are making juices in advance and have a centrifugal juicer you can store for around 12 – 24 hours in the refrigerator. If you have a masticating juicer, then store for 3 days' maximum. Basically the longer you store your juice the more flavour and nutrient content is lost. If you must store juice, then use an airtight sealed container and drink as soon as possible. I often freeze juices immediately after juicing, this way less oxidation and nutrient loss occurs. Try making miniature ice cube juice pops for a healthy summer treat.

Choosing the Best Juicer

There are three types of juicers from which you can choose:

- **Centrifugal**
- **Single gear (masticating)**
- **Twin gear (triturating)**

For most people price is the number one consideration, but several other factors are important.

- Look for an easy-to-use juicer that requires the least effort and time to operate and clean.

- A juicer with at least 0.5 horsepower will not be as easy to burn out.

- Multi-speed mixers are a good investment and will handle more types of produce.

You want a unit that is easy to clean, quiet and stable in operation and versatile in its functions. Look for a juicer that has a large feeding tube and a good sized output.

Always read reviews about the machine and buy a reliable model and brand. Personally I use an Omega Masticating Juicier – I've owned a number of juicers before and this one really suits me (It's particularly easy to clean and very solid)

The Three Types of Juicers

Centrifugal juicers are the least expensive and the least versatile. They are suitable for users who juice on occasion and provide slightly less in terms of nutritional output from the produce. They represent the long end option. I started with one of these juicers, as a starter machine it was great, but my increasingly demanding juicing schedule required a more robust juicer.

Twin gear juicers are at the other end of the spectrum and are best for those with more time, money or those with serious health conditions. These units are versatile, functional, and durable, but can be quite expensive.

A single gear or masticating juicer offers the best combination of benefits for the price:

- **High juice output**
- **Good extraction of nutritional value**
- **Appropriate for grass juicing**
- **Versatile functions**

The features in these units will also allow you to make many things other than juices, including nut butters, sorbet, and baby food.

Masticating juicers squeeze the produce through the gear and then through a fine strainer. The machine does not produce heat or friction so the nutrients are completely preserved.

Remember two key tips to extend the life of your juicer. Remove the pits and cut the fruits or vegetables into small pieces before juicing. This ensures a smooth and quick juicing process and helps the machine to operate with greater efficiency.

Also, clean and wash the juicer and its various parts right after usage. This makes cleaning much easier and ensures the juicer is safe to use next time. Failing to clean your juicer can allow the growth of harmful bacteria.

The Importance of Organic Juices

Using organic produce is one of the most important components of healthy, responsible juicing. As much as possible opt for organic produce from a local source to ensure the highest quality and to avoid harmful toxins.

Modern agricultural methods depend on the heavy use of chemicals. Of the total volume of pesticides and herbicides applied to crops, just 2% kills insects. The remaining 98% penetrates into the soil, air, water and the produce itself. This means that inorganic fruits and vegetables have absorbed high toxic content.

Organic produce is grown without chemicals or pesticides. The strict management process works to restore and to maintain ecological balance. When shopping, look for labels that say "certified" organic. There are strict regulatory standards in place.

Farms and processing facilities are subject to inspection, and soil and water tested. Without these precautions, food cannot carry an organic certified label. Some labels read "transitional organic." This means the produce was grown on a farm that has recently switched to or is switching to organic farming practices.

The produce most likely contaminated by chemicals and pesticides are:

- Strawberries
- Apples
- Apricots
- Peaches
- Cherries
- Grapes
- Celery
- Bell peppers
- Spinach
- Cucumbers
- Green beans

Try and buy organic if you can for these items

If your local supermarket doesn't carry organic produce, try health food stores or a farmer's market. Wash all produce and remove all blemishes and bruises. The skin of the following items can be juiced with the skin on but might alter the taste significantly so take care and try a little first.

- Oranges
- Bananas

- Kiwi fruits
- Pineapples
- Grapefruits
- Tangerines
- Avocados

For most produce it is safe and even advisable to leave on the skins, stems and leaves on since they contain high nutrient content.

Worried About the Taste?

When it comes to the taste of the juice you extract, your own food preferences are crucial determinants. If you have a sweet tooth, then you might prefer adding more fruit with your vegetables.

Keep in mind that not all fruit juices are sweet and not all vegetable juices lack sweetness. Pay more attention to your nutritional requirements rather than the taste. If you find the flavour unpalatable, which can be the case with dark leafy veggies, you can use herbs and fruits to make it more appealing.

Make good use of your taste buds and your creativity to come up with more pleasant tasting and flavoursome combinations.

Chapter 3 - Selection Time

The average daily recommended amount of water for an adult is eight 8-ounce glasses, about 64 fluid ounces. A pregnant woman should add 8 ounces for each hour of light activity daily. All fluids count toward the total amount. Without adequate fluids you may be left feeling dehydrated and lacking in energy.

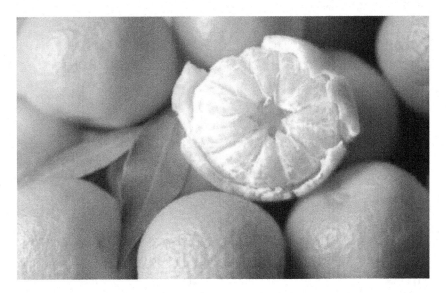

Fruits for Juicing

As an added complication, pregnancy stimulates food cravings that water just won't quench. It's tempting to reach for something full of sugars, preservatives, and chemicals. But if you do, just remember your baby "eats" the same thing.

Juicing creates a satisfying answer for cravings that protects both you and your child from poor nutrition. Eating, juicing and making smoothies can be especially good for this purpose and the following are excellent choices.

Avocados

Avocados are very high in folic acid, a B vitamin, which can help prevent birth defects in the brain and spinal cord. It also plays an important role in making red blood cells.

Pregnant women should include folic acid as a prenatal supplement for at least a month before conceiving, if possible.

Folic acid is essential in the first 3-4 weeks after conceiving. Avocados have 30% of the daily-recommended level of fibre to help lower cholesterol. WOW. True super foods. I eat 1-2 avocados every day – they're just bursting with goodness.

I eat avocados whole, as a daytime snack, remember you don't need to worry about the high fat content in an avocado as its "good fat" and works in an entirely different way to harmful fats. Avocados are also fantastic blended – like most soft fruits they cannot be juiced. For this you will need to use a blender or food processor.

Here's one of my favorite, simple recipes. I have yet to find anyone who doesn't adore this combination.

Babies Delight: Creamy Avocado and Banana Smoothie

1 handful of spinach
½ avocado (de-stoned and peeled)
1 banana
2 cups (480mls) of filtered water

Blended together you will see that avocados and banana really are perfect partners in health crime. Delicious and full of fibre, good fats and a host to a superior blend of pregnancy related micronutrients including vitamin C, B, K and potassium.

HINT: I spread this on toast with a squeeze of fresh lemon or lime (minus the water of course). DELICIOUS

Mangoes

Mangoes are one of the healthiest and most flavourful fruits. They are rich in Vitamin C, polyphenols, beta-carotene, and fibre and one of the best for folate. These nutrients strengthen the immune system and reduce the damage caused by environmental toxins. Mango juice is also excellent for pregnant women experiencing digestive issues and AMAZING for morning sickness, even better if you add ginger.

MORNING MANGO – ANTI-SICKNESS

½" Ginger (juiced or grated into the smoothie)
1 mango (blended)
1 handful spinach (blended)
2 cups (480mls) of filtered water (or more if you prefer a thinner consistency)

Grapes

It is a myth that grapes are harmful for pregnant women. Alcohol is off limits, but grapes are an excellent source of powerful antioxidants. They are full of Vitamin C, Vitamin K, beta-carotene, potassium, sodium, magnesium, and phosphorous.

As an added benefit, grapes don't have a dramatic effect on blood sugar. Grapes are generally great in that they are very low on the glycemic index.

You can blend these, but personally I find they make fantastic snacking.

HINT: Try freezing grapes for a cold, soothing treat throughout the day (the cold can also help take your mind off the aches and pains...)

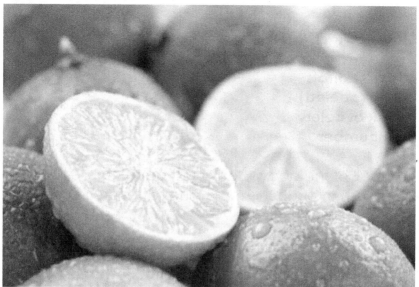

Lime

Limes have more Vitamin C than oranges or lemons. The acidity in the juice helps to relieve nausea and morning sickness during the first trimester of pregnancy. Sometimes all you need to drive away queasiness first thing in the day is a glass of lime juice.

I usually start the day with a glass of warm water with a lemon or a lime. I also add them to the majority of my vegetable juice for a perfect tang – fantastic with green juices if you find them a little bitter.

During pregnancy, including limes will be great for reducing swollen feet and at combating constipation and indigestion - your baby will also benefit from its high potassium level, encouraging the growth of both nerve and brain cells. Here's an easy and very popular juice.

LIMES FOR EINSTEIN'S

4 large carrots
1 lime (peeled)
1 stick of celery
½ cucumber

Juice all of the above, leaving a carrot to use last to help push through the remaining softer produce.

Bananas

Constipation can be an issue at any stage during pregnancy. A smoothie made from an average banana, which has 3 grams of fibre, offers an easy cure. Bananas are also an excellent source of Vitamin C, Vitamin B6, carotenoids, and potassium. As mentioned above, absolutely amazing with avocados.

HINT: I often freeze my bananas, particularly when they are ripe, brown and speckled. Break them up and put them into a small bag or container. Fantastic for a quick morning smoothie.

Oranges

Oranges are one of nature's great multivitamins. They contain Vitamin C, Vitamin A, antioxidants, flavonoids, potassium, calcium, magnesium, folate, and fibre. As an added plus, the sweet, tangy favor helps stop cravings. Eat these whole or juice a few together for the perfect simple fresh orange juice.

Apple

Apple juice is rich in fibre, iron and is a natural cure for heartburn and acidity. They are also rich in Vitamin C and antioxidants, plus a single apple is just 100 calories with no fat. They strengthen the immune system and aid in digestion.

HINT: I always add at least 1 apple to every juice I make. I really do believe the saying "an apple a day....."

Vegetables for Juicing

Vegetables are as important as fruits, but cooking destroys much of their nutritional value. Juicing preserves the full benefit of these foods in a form that is much easier to digest and assimilate. Fruits are easy to eat, but you'll struggle to eat as many whole vegetables as your body requires, particularly during pregnancy. Can you imagine eating a bunch of carrots, a whole cucumber, 3 apples, 2 celery sticks and a whole beetroot all at once? No, but I bet you can imagine the incredible health benefits of juicing these and delivering the goodness straight into your bodies!

Celery

Celery supports efficient digestion and will have a calming effect on your body and baby. Thanks to high levels of potassium, it's also good for the regulation of blood pressure. Celery also stimulates the kidneys to encourage the flushing of uric acid, which can lead to gout. This is a potential problem during pregnancy and a painful one!

HINT: **Fantastic for water retention. Try adding just 1 celery stick to your juice (more if you love the taste. To be honest, I'm not keen – but that doesn't stop me as I want to reap the benefits, I'm just selective in what I juice with the celery)**

DIGESTION HEAVEN

4 large carrots
½ cucumber
2 celery sticks
1 apple

If you're not so keen on the taste of celery juice, then try adding a lime to the equation. I've tried it and it works.

Carrot

My absolute favorites. I juice EVERY **DAY** and I would encourage you to do the same. Seriously, I could write a whole book on these beauties. Carrots are bursting with carotenoids which have been linked to a decrease in a variety of different cancers including

---

bladder, prostate, colon, and breast cancer. You will find carrots in almost all of my RAW juice recipes.

I'm sure you've heard that Carrots are great for eyesight. They are also pretty adept at and cleansing the liver. Carrot juice contains Vitamins A and E. Both are beneficial for the growth of your baby's hair, nails and skin.

Pregnant women can be prone to thyroid problems – the cleansing nature of RAW vegetable juicing; particularly carrots can help to reduce this risk.

HINT: **If you decide to feed breast milk then your baby will also be drinking your vitamin A enriched breast milk.**

Cucumber

Cucumber is rich in Vitamin A, Vitamin C, potassium, sulfur and chlorine. It is also the only vegetable that contains more than 96% water to aid with hydration. Make sure not to peel off the outer skin of the cucumber - it contains the greatest number of nutrients.

Cucumbers are renowned for their skin tightening properties, including these should help address the elasticity issues of your ever expanding belly, possibly helping to reduce cellulite as well.

Recipes

Ok, let's have a look at a few more recipes. With all my clients I try and work on a very individual basis. I look at the system as a whole, specific preferences and personal history. In this book I've included some general recipes, but remember just feel free to add in any other vegetable from the book. **Don't be afraid to experiment.**

That's what I love about juicing; you really can't ever go wrong. If you're experiencing a particularly bad bout of morning sickness, then just add more ginger to your morning juices, do you have particularly swollen feet? – just add more celery.

COOL AS A CARROT

½ cucumber
1 cup spinach
2 stalks of celery
3 carrots
1 apple
1 lime

No blender is required for this recipe, just your favorite juicer.

Juice the cucumber and lime first, followed by the harder vegetables. I always leave a couple of carrots until the end; it helps to push through the softer produce.

Not only will this juice be fantastic for your skin, you will minimize your bloat and load your bodies with the amazing benefits of beta-carotene inside and out.

THE GREEN SPIRITED BABY

1 inch of ginger
½ cucumber
1 handful of spinach
1 lemon
1 celery stick
¼ fennel
2 Apples
6 kale leaves
1 lime

Juice all the ingredients. The juice might look unattractive, but it is bound to energize you and your baby faster than Popeye's spinach and just tastes delicious.

THE ACID SOOTHER

1 large handful spinach
1 celery stick
1 cucumber

Juice the three ingredients. The acidic properties of these combined will counteract your digestive upset and provide a refreshing juice. Remember, cucumber isn't just cooling; it contains Folic acid so will help protect you against anemia.

Fruits and Vegetables to avoid when pregnant

Fruits and vegetables are beneficial, high nutrient

foods, but not all will be suitable for a pregnant woman.

Pineapples

Pineapple contains large amounts of bromelain. Usually this is a fantastic trait. However, this enzyme can cause softening of the cervix and possibly lead to premature labour during pregnancy if eaten in excess. By excess, I mean more than a few pineapples a day, which might be a hard job unless of course you happen to be craving pineapples.

Avoid eating or drinking larger amounts during the first trimester, after this then smaller amounts can be tolerated more easily.

Papaya

Papayas will help you to control heartburn, constipation and are rich in vitamin C.

However, you need to make sure the papaya is very ripe - as an unripe or semi-ripe papaya contains latex, this can cause uterine contractions and possibly an early labour.

Some expecting mothers avoid it altogether; personally I believe you will gain lots of health benefits from eating ripe papaya.

RAW Vegetables

Avoid eating RAW vegetables like radish, alfalfa and

clover. They are rich in listeria causing bacteria. It is always better to rinse these items, and/or cook them before you eat them.

Washing produce is a "best practice" to protect against bacteria. Unwashed fruits and vegetables are home to a parasite called "toxoplasma" which can cause "toxoplasmosis" this disease is very dangerous to unborn children and can also be found in the faces of infected cats.

Herbs for Juicing

For centuries, healers used herbal remedies for simple and even life-threatening illness. Regarded now as "folk" medicine, many of these plants are helpful during pregnancy. Use the following herbs daily in your juices to maximize your nutritional intake.

Ginger

It's not a fruit, it's not a veg. It's a WONDERFULLY zingy, aromatic and a truly amazing herb.

I try and include ginger every day in my juices, smoothies or my cooked meals. You simply cannot have too much. Your immune system will really thank you for this.

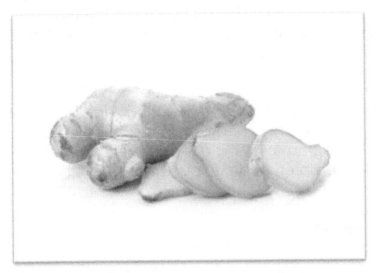

There are numerous medicinal uses for ginger and if you can stomach the spiciness, it does wonders in treating many disorders including nausea and morning sickness. Try just one teaspoonful with some honey – this should really help in alleviating these symptoms, also fantastic for dizziness and nausea caused by chemotherapy or anesthesia.

My favorite juice containing lots of ginger juice is my....

MORNING GINGER ZINGER

1/3 " Ginger
1 apple
3 carrots
½ lemon
½ lime

Zingy, tangy and just AMAZING.

HOMEMADE GINGER ALE

This juice is a tasty chilled treat and it's easy to make. If you're in need of something warm whether you're pregnant or not, then gently heat 2 gallons of water and add a tablespoon of grated or freshly juiced ginger.

Allow the mixture to cool. Juice four lemons and add the liquid to the mixture – if you are not sensitive to yeast, or trying to omit it for health reasons then ass ¼ teaspoon. Set aside for two days until the mixture takes on a shiny, crystal glaze, then refrigerate and keep chilled for drinking.

Yam/ Sweet potato

Wild yam / sweet potatoes have wondrous healing properties, including relieving uterine pain. It also helps to calm the nerves and acts as a remedy for nausea. Almost all women experience some cramping during pregnancy. Wild yams help to ease those pains and can help to prevent miscarriage.

The juice is so sweet; you can juice this on its own or add cucumber and parsley for a perfect combination.

Although Yam / Sweet potatoes come from the same family – Yams are a little less moist so more may be required.

YUMMY MUMMY YAM-YAM JUICE

2 small yams / sweet potatoes
2 carrots
¼ inch Ginger
1 apple
Small handful parsley
1 lemon
½ cucumber

Red Raspberry

Not only does this amazing fruit promote rapid healing it also provides relief from labour pains and can help to regulate bleeding during delivery. Both the leaves and fruit are effective. After your baby is born, red raspberry increases and purifies milk production. Try to drink at least one cup per day throughout your pregnancy. This will help pain generally, whether its labour pains, aches, nipple pain from breast feeding or general postnatal pain.

Raspberries are also known as very efficient cancer fighters, containing ellagic acid which can slow some tumor growths.

Try this delicious smoothie for an effective super healing, pain reducing treat.

RASPBERRY NIPPLE

1 banana
2 handfuls of raspberries (fresh or frozen)
1 cup (240mls) filtered water
½ - 1 teaspoon honey

Place all ingredients into your blender for roughly 30 seconds or until desired consistency is reached – add more water if required.

A Few Things to Remember

As a pregnant mother natural juices offer the ideal form of nutrient intake. Before you begin to juice, talk with your obstetrician. As you begin to design your juice drinks try and include as much variety as possible. The fruits, vegetables, and herbs you use should contain the correct balance of:

- Vitamins
- Minerals
- Protein
- Fatty acids
- Carbohydrates
- Calcium
- Potassium

Make juicing vegetables and herbs your priority – remember it's easier to eat your fruit. The sugar in fruit, when combined with soluble fibre, increases blood sugar, so keep fruit to a minimum when using in juices/smoothies.

TIP: Alkaline content of vegetables will combat toxic waste in your system. If you do drink fruit juice, do so early in the day. Avoid mixing fruit juice with meals and try to drink a fresh juice as soon as you wake up.

This might all feel a bit overwhelming, ultimately don't worry too much – juice and enjoy it. One juice a day is better than no juice.

Chapter 4 - Make the Most of Juicing

As I'm sure you will have gathered by now, juicing during pregnancy is not about picking up a can of juice at the grocery store. It can be hard work – but you will both benefit greatly. Once you make it part of the daily routine it really becomes as easy as making a fresh cup of coffee or changing nappies.

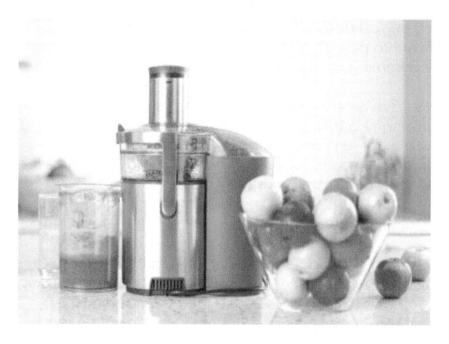

There are some common mistakes that are crucial you avoid.

Common Juicing Mistakes

The "big three" mistakes of juicing are taking in too

---

much sugar, gulping, and buying prepared juices at the store.

Adding Excessive Amounts of Sugar

One common misconception is that unless you use fruit, you won't enjoy the taste of your juices. Fruit contains large quantities of fructose or sugar, which are difficult for the liver to metabolize.

When you combine fruits and vegetables, you create juices full of nutrients and fibre in an easy to digest form. You don't want to exclude fruits, but you do want to pay attention to the amount of sugar you are consuming.

Don't overdo it. As mentioned in the previous chapter, juicing vegetables is your priority. I do however tend to use 1 apple in every juice because they are so incredibly good for you and have a mild sweetness I enjoy. I also eat apples most days.

Gulping Down Your Juice

Gulping down a full glass is not a healthy way to consume fresh juice; you are likely to create various stomach related issues. Take the time to enjoy the juice, especially if it contains fruit, so you will be less likely to cause an instant spike in your blood sugar. Be mindful and give your stomach time to do a proper job of digesting what you're taking in. Enjoy your hard work...take small sips and relax...

Buying Pasteurized and Preserved Juices

Don't let bottled juices tempt you.

They do not offer you the same level of nutritional benefit as fresh juice and may contain harmful preservatives. Always remember, you and your child deserve the best.

Preparation Advice

For the most part, juicing is a simple process. Still, there are a few tips and tricks to make it even easier and more effective.

- **Wash all fruits and vegetables to make sure they are free of pesticides and bacteria. You only need to rinse if you have bought organic produce.**

- **Line the walls of your pulp basket with a bag to make cleaning up faster and easier.**

- **Cut your produce into small pieces, but wait until you are ready to put them into the machine. Once sliced, fruits and vegetables instantly begin to lose their nutritional value.**

- **Adjust the juicer speed to match the produce you are processing. Apples and beets, for instance, need a higher processing speed, as opposed to spinach and lettuce.**

If you think that your pulp is thick, even after passing it through your machine, then re-juice it. Re-processing squeezes out the remaining moisture and softens the consistency of your juice.

Tips for Storing Juice

During pregnancy, it is hard enough to move a muscle, let alone drag yourself into the kitchen every morning to make fresh juice.

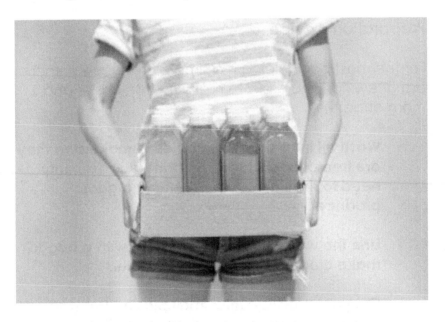

You can make double batches and refrigerate them for later use, but do not store juice longer than a day unless you have a masticating juicer – if you do, 3 days is acceptable.

Use an air tight container filled to the brim. Oxygen in the container lessens the nutritional value of your ingredients. If you freeze juice, use it within 10 days.

Buying Quality Produce

Washing your produce is your best defense against bacteria and contaminants. Buying organic protects you from pesticides and other chemicals. But how do you determine the quality of the produce you select?

Buy only ripe fruits and vegetables. Otherwise, you will face unpleasant digestive issues. Be careful that there are no black, rotten spots on the produce. If blemishes are present, cut away those parts before juicing.

- **Apples should have smooth skin and a firm feel with a full, rich color.**

- **Look for berries that are plump and firm with a uniform color and no dullness. Ripe blueberries have a powdery white coating called "bloom." This is normal and desirable.**

- **Grapes should be firm and plump with tight attachment at the stems. Also look for a uniform color regardless of the variety of grape.**

- **With citrus fruit, including lemons and oranges, look for heavy weight in relation to size with vibrant color.**

- **Celery stalks should be about 8 inches long. They should be firm, green glossy, and have a fresh aroma.**

- **Mature carrots are roughly a half inch in diameter, with a bright color, firm body, and smooth skin. The leaves should be crisp and a**

healthy green.

- **Cucumbers should be a rich, dark green. The body should by heavy, firm, and about 6 inches in length.**

If you're unsure about the produce just ask the green grocer for help.

Quality of Utensils

Before you start juicing, make sure your juicer is clean, with no remnants stuck near the metal fan. You can avoid this by filling your juicer with soaped, lukewarm water that you allow to stand for 10 minutes after every use. Also be sure to use a clean glass and utensils each time.

"Extras" to take Your Juice up a Level

To stick with juicing, you need to enjoy what you're drinking. Take your juices and smoothies up to another level of taste with some of the following ingredients:

Cacao

Cacao is RAW chocolate, which is rich in phenethylamine to help your focus and attention. An occasional tablespoon of cacao in your morning smoothie can give you an instant boost of energy, which will last throughout the day.

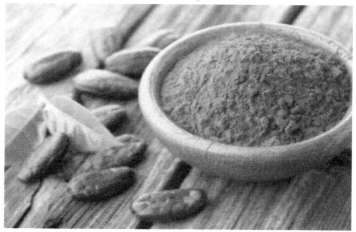

RAW cacao will benefit you in a number of different ways. As well as containing essential B vitamins and high amounts of iron you will find potassium, manganese, copper, zinc, calcium, and magnesium. It's a true super food! Cacao is also really useful to anyone trying to eat a lower cholesterol, lower fat diet.

Cacao beans are the purest form available, but cacao powder is more convenient for mixing in juices and smoothies. I usually recommend around 1-2 tablespoons, however some people are a little more sensitive to cacao, so if you find yourself feeling a little too alert then recue to 1 tablespoon.

TIP: You can also purchase RAW cacao nibs, I like to sprinkle these either on my smoothies, breakfast porridge or eat as a snack.

Goji-Berries

Goji-berries are the most natural form of plant-based protein. They are rich in beta-carotene and provide an instant energy boost. Use the berries in their dry, RAW state. They are absolutely delicious when used in conjunction with cacao.

Maca

Maca is a root vegetable indigenous to Peru. It increases stamina and is useful during the last trimester of pregnancy. Buy RAW maca, not the powder or tablets. Use about 3 tablespoons in your juice or the taste may be overpowering. Avoid over-consumption to avoid thyroid-related problems.

Chia

Chia seeds are an excellent source of Omega 3, which supports the development of the baby's nervous system and vision. Omega-3s also protect the unborn child from the development of future allergy. For the mother, Omega 3s prevent premature labour, pre-eclampsia, and postpartum depression.

Give the seeds a thorough rinse and let them sit for 10 minutes in water.

Note that if you have high estrogen levels, you may need to avoid chia seeds.

Below are some of my favorite recipes using these amazing super foods – most of these I include when I make my detox juices and 3-day juicing detox plans due to the high quantity and quality of the natural ingredients.

GOOD MORNING MACA

1 banana- frozen or fresh
2 pitted Medjool date
1 tbs Maca powder
1 tbs Cacao nibs
1 cup (240mls) of almond milk
½ cup (120mls) coconut milk
Coconut flakes and/or Cacao nibs for sprinkling

Blend the ingredients in a food processor. Control the speed until you achieve a smooth consistency. Sprinkle the smoothie with coconut flakes and cacao nibs for extra garnish and serve chilled.

GOGI, MACA and CACAO SMOOTHIE

1 banana- fresh or frozen, whichever is available
1 cup (240mls) coconut or almond milk
1 small handful Goji berries
1 tbs Maca powder
1 tbs Cacao powder
1 handful blueberries- fresh or frozen
<u>Extra Ingredients</u> (Super Foods):
1 tsp Bee pollen
1 tsp Coconut Oil

Blend all ingredients; super foods are optional. Keep the blender on for about 30-45 seconds or until the consistency is correct.

SUPER GREEN SMOOTHIE

1 handful Goji Berries
1 tsp chia seeds
¼ glass of filtered water
1 banana (Frozen or ripe)
1 handful of seasonal fruit
1 handful of green leafy vegetables- Mint, Chard & Spinach
1 tsp coconut oil

Blend all ingredients at medium speed. Add cold coconut oil and ice cubes to chill the smoothie to make it super refreshing.

AVOCADO & MACA SMOOTHIE

1 handful of berries (any type of berry will do)
1 frozen banana
4 Medjool pitted dates
Water, Soy Milk or Almond Milk- 1 cup
½ Avocado
1 tsp Maca Root Powder
1 tsp Vanilla Extract

Blend all the ingredients to the desired consistency.

Prenatal Vitamin Juices

Prenatal vitamins support conception, pregnancy, and lactation. The formulas are rich in vitamins and minerals essential for mother and child like folic acid, iron, and calcium. Available in liquid, tablet, and pill form, prenatal vitamins can carry unpleasant side effects:

- insomnia
- headaches
- cramps
- indigestion
- acidity
- nausea
- sluggishness
- urinary problems
- muscle aches

Pregnant women require roughly 1000 mg of calcium, 30 mg of iron and 600 mcgs of folic acid daily. Juices designed to meet these needs can be a more palatable and nutritious way of meeting these needs. Items rich in folic acid, for instance, include:

- strawberries
- lettuce
- spinach
- citrus fruits

Some great prenatal juices include:

GINGER PEACH PASSION

2 peaches
½ teaspoon of grated ginger,
¼ cup diced mango
1 cup (240mls) of filtered water.

(Substitute coconut water if you like, or a cup of low fat yogurt.)

Blend the ingredients and enjoy!

BANANA & APRICOT FREEZE

½ cup (120mls) of almond milk
½ cup (120mls) of low fat live yogurt
1 banana
1 small handful of apricots

Bananas are high in vitamins and potassium that support good energy. Apricots are rich in Vitamins A, K, C and E, and provide dietary fibre. Blend all the ingredients and enjoy.

GRAPEFRUIT, CARROT & GINGER JUICE

2 grapefruits
5 carrots
1 inch of fresh ginger.

Combine the ingredients and stir well.

This juice serves as a great detoxifier, packed with essential prenatal nutrients. Grapefruit contains high levels of Vitamin A and C, potassium, fibre, folate and lycopene.

Juicing and Pregnancy FAQs

Some of the most frequent questions asked about juicing during pregnancy include the following.

Why is juicing better than eating?

Drinking, rather than eating fruits and vegetables allows for greater quantities consumed. Often, cooking vegetables extracts most of their nutritional value. Juicing RAW vegetables preserves the full dose of the vitamins and minerals. Research indicates juicing helps high blood pressure, various skin disease and even certain cancers.

Why is juicing better for digestion?

Digesting liquids, as opposed to solids, is easier for you as well as your baby. It takes less energy to digest RAW vegetables and fruits, reducing fatigue.

Are all juices equal?

NO. Not all types of juices are healthy.
RAW forms are usually the ones with the greatest number of minerals and vitamins. Packaged and pasteurized juices are usually high in sugar, which can be harmful for the mother, as well as the baby.

What are the various methods of juicing?

You can extract juice from fruits and vegetables by hand, or with a juicer or blender. Centrifugal juicing uses a spinning meal blade to grind fruits and vegetables. Masticating uses a motor for grinding and blending. Triturating juicers use more than one gear and are faster and more durable.

How many calories should there be in your juice?

You can't pinpoint the ideal combination of calories in your juice. It will vary from person to person. You honestly don't need to carefully consider calories when juicing, it's RAW, fat-free and it's great for you – it's REALLY all you need to know.

Should I juice to the exclusion of eating?

No. The trick is to maintain a balance between eating and juicing. The most effective way to do this is by apportioning parts of the day to each activity. Allot mornings for juicing and eat healthy vegetables for dinner. You can also add a bit of pulp to your juices, so that you and your baby get a fair share of fibre intake.

Chapter 5 - Pregnancy and Nutrition

Start making healthy dietary choices three months to a year before conception. Research has shown that nutrition plays a significant role in fertility for both men and women. All the following should be present in your diet.

Folic Acid

Folic acid reduces the risk of neural tube birth defects including spina bifida. You should have at least 400 micrograms (0.4 milligrams) of this B vitamin daily. Folic Acid is found in all green leafy vegetables, citrus fruits, nuts, legumes and whole grains.

Magnesium

Magnesium helps to build and repair tissues. During pregnancy a deficiency can cause poor fetal growth, preeclampsia, and even affect infant mortality. Increased levels will also help to prevent premature uterine contractions.

Magnesium builds teeth and bones, regulates insulin and blood sugar, and improves enzyme function. It may also help control cholesterol, heart arrhythmia, and leg cramps. Pregnant women benefit from 310-400 mg per day.

Zinc

The body needs zinc to build and repair DNA, a crucial support for rapid cell growth during pregnancy. Zinc supports the immune system, maintains the sense of taste and smell, and heals wounds. A deficiency can lead to miscarriage, toxemia, and low birth weight among other problems. Pregnant women benefit from 11-14 mg a day.

Vitamin B12

Vitamin B12 with folic acid offers more effective protection against neural tube birth defects. The recommended daily dose is 400 micrograms.

Omega 3

Omega 3 supports fetal neurological and visual development. Pregnant women can become deficient because the baby uses the nutrient for the nervous system development. After birth, Omega 3s are important for breast milk production. Some studies believe Omega 3s also protect infants against developing allergies.

Start planning your nutritional needs as soon as you learn you're pregnant. You will need more calories to have the energy you need to carry your baby and to help your child develop.

Try to aim for roughly: -

70 grams of protein per day
45-60% daily calories from carbohydrates
No more than 35% daily calories from fat

The following recipes are not only rich in the recommended nutrients but will give you an instant boost of energy.

BABY BEET JUICE

Beetroot has strong antioxidant content, as well as fibre and vitamins. Some research indicates beet juice increases fertility. It is also boosts iron content and helps purify the blood.

2 apples
½ RAW beetroot
4 carrots
1 cup (240mls) filtered water

Juice all the ingredients and add filtered water to the desired consistency, separate the pulp from the juice with a strainer. Add ice if required and serve chilled.

CUCUMBER REFRESHER

Cucumbers contains "feel good" B vitamins. Cucumbers work wonders for the skin, tightening, lightening and enhancing.

1 unpeeled cucumber
½ medium melon (any will do)
½ lemon

½ cup filtered water

Mix all ingredients in a blender, using water to smooth the consistency. Add ice and serve.

HOT GINGER ZINGER

Ginger works well for vomiting and nausea, soothing the stomach, and improving digestion. (Ginger also eases the pain and aches of inflamed joints.)

1 inch piece of ginger
1 apple
4 carrots
1 celery stick
1 cucumber
1 lime

Smooth, spicy and delicious.

Chapter 6 - Dealing with Pregnancy Related Issues

Being energetic and pregnant doesn't have to be a contradictory state. Fatigue is normal, but you can lessen its effects. Good nutrition is the key to good energy, sharp focus and concentration.

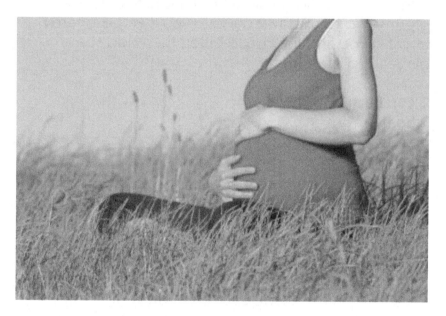

Combating Fatigue

Your body makes huge changes to carry your unborn child. It works hard to create the placenta, which is the baby's life-support system. Your metabolism changes, your hormone levels fluctuate, and blood sugar and pressure are lower. These changes all contribute to feeling tired.

You need your five daily servings of fruits and vegetables, but keeping food down may be a problem. Most pregnant women deal with this by eating several small meals a day. Juicing makes this task MUCH easier, and offers a much better, highly concentrated dose of vitamins and minerals.

CAULIFLOWER & BROCCOLI JUICE

Vitamin B and magnesium from the broccoli, beet greens and cauliflower will give you a HUGE energy boost. If you find this a little bitter, then add some ginger and an apple.

1 cup fresh cauliflower
2 beet greens
4 broccoli spears
1 lemon

Juice each vegetable alone, then combine the juice for a potent, tasty and chemical free energy drink.

POPEYE PICKER-UPPER

Watercress is excellent for anemia and is full of pregnancy supportive nutrients. These include iron, calcium, iodine, folic acid, Vitamin C and Vitamin A.

1 apple
2 handfuls of watercress
1 handful of spinach leaves
½ inch fresh ginger

Juice together and serve at room temperature or

chilled – which ever you prefer, just don't leave it too long...

BANANA BLISS SMOOTHIE

A mix of apple and banana helps increase your energy levels and also helps in combating anemia. Apples are high in Vitamin C and bananas are rich in Vitamin C, B6, manganese, potassium, fibre, biotin, and copper.

2 apples (preferably Granny Smith or Braeburn)
2 large handfuls of fresh blackberries
1 lemon
1 banana

Juice the apples and lemon and then blend the mixture together with the blackberries and banana. You can't not LOVE this combination

Morning Sickness

Morning sickness, which may include nausea and vomiting is unfortunately very common. For some of you it may last throughout your pregnancy, hopefully it'll be the average of a few weeks (fingers crossed....)

Although you're more likely to wake up in the morning feeling sick, the nausea and vomiting can occur at any time during the day. Smells often trigger the queasy feelings, but fluctuating hormones are the real culprit here.

Morning sickness can prove to be overwhelming for many women. Some doctors regard morning sickness as a psychological condition, but that is far from the truth. The condition can cause severe dehydration sometimes necessitating hospitalization.

To help combat morning sickness eat small light meals or snacks throughout the day. Avoid spicy foods and drink plenty of fluids – even better try these juices...

SUPER CELERY JUICE

**3 apples
3 stalks of celery
1 inch ginger**

This is a fantastic daily juice, many of my clients swear by drinking this immediately upon waking. You could try making it before bedtime and chill in the fridge overnight. DELICIOUS. If the taste of the celery is a little strong, try adding 1 lemon or Lime – or adding additional filtered water.

FEELING FENNEL FANTASTIC

**3 carrots
½ fennel bulb
1 celery stick
1 inch of fresh ginger**

Like ginger, fennel is also useful to reduce nausea and settle the stomach. Celery keeps the body hydrated and flushes out the toxins.

MORNING MELON SMOOTHIE

2 carrots
1 inch of ginger
1 lime
½ Gala or Honeydew melon
1 handful white or red grapes

The lime adds nice flavour and Vitamin C, while the melon is fantastic for hydration.

You can also add some **fresh peppermint** or spearmint. Both soothe the stomach and enhance flavour.

Juice the ginger, lime and carrots – then blend with the melon and grapes.

High Blood Pressure and Pre-Eclampsia

High blood pressure, or hypertension, can lead to serious health problems if left uncontrolled. These include:

- heart attack
- heart failure
- kidney dysfunction
- stroke

People suffering from hypertension may experience

- nausea
- shortness of breath
- restlessness

- headaches

High blood pressure before you are 20 weeks pregnant is pre-existing hypertension. High blood pressure after 20 weeks is gestational hypertension. It will disappear after your child is born and is only rarely a cause for concern.

The following juice recipes are helpful in regulating blood pressure.

NO PRESSURE COCKTAIL

1 apple
2 celery stalks
½ cucumber
4 leaves of kale
1 lemon
2 peeled oranges
Handful of parsley

The high calcium content of celery has a calming effect. Lemon juice contains potassium, which controls blood pressure and soothes nausea. It relaxes the muscles and nerves in the body and mind. Oranges contain the flavonoid hesperidin, which lowers blood pressure.

POWER ME UP JUICE

Juice the following ingredients for a powerful blood pressure-lowering juice.

2 carrots
½ RAW beetroot

2 celery stalks
½ a cucumber
2 handfuls of parsley
½ green bell pepper
1 handful of spinach
3 medium tomatoes

Both celery and spinach lower blood pressure while bell peppers help to reduce cholesterol levels. Beetroot is pretty amazing when it comes to lowering blood pressure – this is due to the high levels of dietary nitrate (NO_3) - which naturally widens blood vessels, therefore lowering blood pressure. I love it and try to drink beetroot most days – if I'm not drinking it then I'm eating it raw.

CALMER KALE JUICE

1 apple
1 small beetroot
1 stalk of celery
1 cucumber
½ lemon
1 inch of ginger
3 large kale leaves

This mixture contains useful quantities of potassium, magnesium and fibre. All are beneficial in treating hypertension.

During pregnancy high blood pressure can also lead to pre-eclampsia. Reduced blood flow to the placenta disrupts the transport of oxygen and nutrients to the baby. Pre-eclampsia occurs most often during the second half of pregnancy or just before delivery.

There are several things you can do to help control your blood pressure and lower your risk for pre-eclampsia. Doctors recommend reduced salt intake, higher levels of protein and a concentration on diuretic foods. My advice is keep juicing....

SWEET BEET

1 large beetroot
½ sweet potato / yam
½ cucumber
4 carrots
1 celery stick
1 apple

Celery calms the nerves and along with the brilliant beetroot is a natural diuretic.

KARMA GREEN

4 carrots
½ beetroot
2 apples
Handful of spinach
3-4 leaves of kale
1 handful of coriander / cilantro
1 Lime

Carrots have strong antioxidant properties, while spinach and kale both lower blood pressure. Coriander has anticoagulant properties, while lemon is a diuretic.

Also consider drinking watermelon juice. Watermelon is rich in Vitamin C, beta-carotene, antioxidants, and lycopene. The taste is pleasant, and watermelon is fantastic for hydration. (You can also try adding small amounts of garlic to your juices for its anticoagulant properties.)

WATER BABY SMOOTHIE

½ watermelon
10 mint leaves
1 orange
1 clove of garlic

Iron Deficiency

Iron deficiency or anemia can potentially be a major pregnancy-related issue. It can affect development and possibly lead to complications both during and after pregnancy.

Lowered hemoglobin production causes anemia. Hemoglobin is a protein in red blood cells that transports oxygen throughout the body. During pregnancy, the need for increased iron rises significantly.

Doctors usually recommend prenatal iron supplements and an iron-rich diet. Unfortunately, constipation is often a side effect of supplementation. Iron-rich foods like red meat, fish, lentils, whole grain bread, green leafy vegetables, and dried fruits are often better options.

And of course the great news is you can also juice to help guard against anemia – not only are these juices fantastic for boosting your iron naturally – they also taste sensational.

THE SPICY IRON

2 cups Swiss chard
1 apple
½ cucumber
1 celery stalk
1 lemon
2 inch ginger root

Apples, Swiss chard and celery are all excellent sources of iron. Leafy green vegetables contain oxalate that help slow iron absorption. The Vitamin C from the lemon neutralizes the oxalates and improves iron absorption in the bloodstream. What more could you want...

IRON WOMAN SUPER GREEN

1 apple
3 carrots
1 beetroot
2 sticks of celery
1 large handful of spinach
2 inch Broccoli
3 tomatoes

Apples, beetroot, celery, spinach, and kale all have plenty of iron content. Carrots lend a good taste to every juice and build the blood by enhancing the hemoglobin production.

In any juice you make to help combat anemia you should aim to include vegetables or fruit with a high Vitamin C content (with low calcium) to improve iron absorption.

Constipation

Unfortunately, over half of pregnant women suffer from constipation; this is defined as fewer than 3 bowel movements per week. Hard, dry stools that are difficult to pass are also common. The major causes are:

- Poor intake of fluid and fibre
- Insufficient exercise
- Raised levels of the hormone progesterone
- Iron and calcium supplements

Progesterone is necessary for the production of the placenta – unfortunately though the side effects can lead to a reduction in the frequency and strength of bowel movements.

Fruits and vegetables that can ease constipation include:

- Apples
- Bananas
- Beets
- Carrots
- Alfalfa sprouts

- Cauliflower
- Peaches
- Pears
- Spinach
- Asparagus
- Cabbage
- Figs
- Papaya

As much as possible try to use purified/filtered water in your smoothies – this will help to prevent hardening of fibre in the intestines.

To help combat constipation, try the following juices.

BOWEL DOWN

Juice the following for an easy drink that aids digestion and works absolute wonders for relieving constipation.

2 pears
½ large pineapple
½ inch of ginger
1 cup (240mls) filtered water

Pears contain pectin, which is a soluble fibre that helps to flush out toxins. The enzyme bromelain in pineapple also aids digestion.

SMOOTH OPERATOR

This juice lives up to its name by relieving constipation and aiding digestion.

4 carrots
3 fresh or re-hydrated figs
1 orange
1 banana
1 inch of ginger

Juice the vegetables together first, then blend together with the banana.

PEAR, SPINACH & PRUNE JUICE

2 pears
2 handfuls of spinach
25 grams pitted prunes
½ cup (240mls) filtered water

Each of these ingredients is well known for their constipation relieving properties.
Drink this for a huge sigh of relief. Prunes truly do work wonders.

CITRUS CUCUMBER COOLER

A natural diuretic and is great for digestion.

1 peeled pink grapefruit
1 peeled orange
1/4 inch of ginger
1 cucumber

The citrus fruits provide vitamin C and enhance the immune system. Cucumber is an excellent source of necessary fluids that lubricate the intestines.

You can also add flaxseed, chia seeds, or psyllium husks to any of these the juices or smoothies for an even more powerful relief of constipation.

Blood Circulation

Blood circulation transports oxygen and essential nutrients throughout the body. Disruptions in the flow can lead to health problems. A pregnant woman's body produces 30% - 50% more blood to adapt to the needs of the unborn baby.

The rise in blood pressure that accompanies the increased volume can cause:

- Swelling in the legs and feet
- Pressure in the veins of the lower part of the body
- Fatigue
- Headaches
- Hemorrhoids
- Improper fetal development
- Pre-eclampsia
- Anemia

For proper circulation, doctors suggest sleeping on the left side. This helps to ensure flow through the vena cava, the major vein to the lower extremities. Also avoid standing for long periods and sit with your feet up.

Here are some delicious juice recipes to help enhance your circulation...

THE CITRUS CIRCULATOR

3 cups (375grams) cranberries
1 inch of ginger root
1 small peeled grapefruit
1 lime
3 oranges
1 Lemon
½ cup (120mls) filtered water

The ginger stimulates circulation, relaxing the muscles around the blood vessels and preventing clots. Flavonoids in the oranges called hesperidin help to lower blood pressure.

GINGER PARADISE

1 apple
4 carrots
½ pineapple
1 cucumber
1 inch of ginger

I adore this one. The carrots and apples assist in blood production, while ginger improves circulation. Pure paradise in a glass....

FULL IMMUNITY ENERGIZER

1 apple
3 carrots
2 cloves of garlic
1 inch ginger root
1 handful of parsley

Ginger enhances circulation. It has warming properties that make it a natural decongestant and immune system booster. Apples and carrots are a fantastic source of iron, and carrots are natural blood builders.

You honestly can't get better than this.

Non-Specific Dermatitis

Non-specific dermatitis is an inflammation of the skin. It can cause red, flaky patches on the face and sometimes the arms. This skin allergy may be due to exposure to environmental substances or as a result of changes to the body brought on by pregnancy.

Whatever the case, these rashes are uncomfortable. The infection is not contagious and is not a cause for worry. However, if it starts to spread, itches, or causes a fever then a medical consultation may be necessary.

Otherwise, you can take care of the condition at home. Keep the area clean. Avoid skin irritants and drink fresh juices and smoothies that have anti-inflammatory properties.

Try and include some of the following, here's some great recipes to get you started.

- Alfalfa
- Lemon
- Ginger
- Celery
- Parsley
- Grapes
- Cucumber
- Spinach
- Beet
- Pear
- Plum

SHINY SKIN JUICE

Choose a handful of ANY green leafy vegetables.

Watercress
Spring greens
Lettuce
Kale
Parsley
Spinach

Then add the following

1 apple
2 carrots
1 stick of celery
½ cucumber
¼ broccoli stem
1 handful of alfalfa sprouts

¼ **inch RAW beetroot**
¼ **inch courgette/zucchini**
1 **lemon**
¼ **inch of ginger**

This juice will boost the immune system and help to fight inflammation; it's also amazing for the skin thanks to high levels of Vitamin A.

RAINBOW BLITZ

1 **apple**
5 **carrots**
½ **cucumber**
1 **inch of ginger root**
1 **lemon**
1 **pear**
2 **handfuls of spinach**

As usual we have the ginger in here to help reduce any inflammation. The alkaline nature of spinach helps heal the rash, as does the pear juice that reduces inflammation and soothes pain.

Breast Milk Issues

Mastitis

Mastitis is a bacterial infection of the breasts and can be very painful. Symptoms include fever, cold, cough, and throbbing pain. Breasts may swell, with cracking of the skin and the milk ducts may also become clogged.

Low Supply of Milk

A lower than usual milk supply is common, especially in first-time mothers. The best way to increase milk production is by aiming to increase your liquid intake as much as possible. Drink as much filtered water as you can - also juices and smoothies that are rich in calories and aim to help support milk supply.

Too Much Milk

On the other end of the spectrum, some women can produce too much milk. This can lead to aches and pains in the breasts, and opens the door for potential infection.

Clogged Ducts

The breasts will be sore with discernible lumps. Long gaps between breast feeding or wearing a nursing bra that is too tight can cause this problem.

You can help to increase the flow of your breast milk by increasing your liquid intake and aiming to juice at least once daily.

These juices are a great start to help in the prevention of painful breasts and in encouraging a healthy milk supply.

THE BETTER BREAST

5 carrots
1 handful of spinach
4 beet leaves
3 asparagus
1 apple
5 basil leaves
2 garlic cloves
2 apricots
1 cup (240mls) filtered water

Carrots work wonders for the breast and contain an array of nutrients to help enhance and promote lactation - in fact, carrots are just absolutely wonderful – full stop. High in vitamin K, A and C, asparagus is an absolute essential when it comes to breast issues – helping to stimulate the hormones that are responsible for lactation.

Try this wonderful juice, great for increasing breast flow, production and overall breast health.

The Pregnancy Mask (Chloasma)

The skin inflammation chloasma or melasma was once thought prevalent in darker skinned women only. Research shows it occurs in 70% of pregnancies. The dark spots or patches of abnormal pigmentation look like a mask across the nose, forehead and cheeks. This is generally caused by hormonal fluctuations that make take 2-3 months to resolve.

The following is a fantastic natural treatment that can

help to normalize and nourish your skin. I haven't tried this one myself but my clients tell me it works wonders.

MAGIC MASK MIX

1 tsp RAW Apple Cider Vinegar
1 tsp RAW honey
1 tsp fresh lemon juice
2 tsp horseradish
1 tsp almond oil
1 ripe banana
1 teaspoon filtered water

Mix all the ingredients in a bowl until you have a smooth mixture. Apply as a paste to the pigmented areas. Allow the treatment to dry for 10-15 minutes. Rinse with water and a soft, damp cloth.

You can also try mashing a banana and adding RAW honey to form a paste. Apply in the same fashion and leave in place for 20-25 minutes. Wash your face with lukewarm water and pat your skin dry.

(Actually I have to be honest this sounds very tasty too!)

Depression and Anxiety

Otherwise known as the 'Baby Blues' - roughly 30% of women suffer anxiety and depression during or after pregnancy. Raging hormones in the body can be a common cause; however, a range of factors can come into play.

In the majority of cases these feelings are totally

normal – usually reducing in their intensity over the coming weeks.

However, in some cases symptoms manifest in clinical postnatal depression and this can be overwhelming and distressing– if symptoms increase in intensity, if you are having unusual or distressing thoughts, feeling hopeless or feel your anxiety is excessive then you must contact your medical practitioner for further advice or assessment. This can be a serious clinical condition that with support will resolve.

Fertility

If you have received fertility treatments to conceive you are also at a higher risk for stress during pregnancy. Fear of losing a child under such circumstances if high. Anxious mothers understandably can exhaust themselves with hypervigilance and worry. Try and use mindfulness and relaxation techniques as much as possible, this can be so beneficial and help promote healing in all dimensions.

Hereditary

Some families have generational problems with anxiety and depression. Pregnancy can aggravate those tendencies. If you are afraid this may be the case, you can try to take measure to deal with the issues before they occur, be mindful in relation to changes and seek support from appropriate agencies and professionals.

Relationship Blues

Although the arrival of a new baby is an exciting time - changing dynamics can naturally cause stress. If you are feeling stressed and anxious before your baby arrives, seek counseling. Be as open as possible – try not make the mistake of thinking the arrival of the baby will fix everything. You want to welcome your child into a happy, satisfied situation. A relaxed and loving parent or parents is all any child could hope for.

Past Miscarriages

Past miscarriages can have a profound effect on mental and emotional well-being. It is only natural to carry a certain anxiety into a new pregnancy.

Specific Pregnancy Problems

Not all pregnancies are healthy and trouble free; some pose a higher risk to the mother and the baby alike. If you must undergo strenuous tests and procedures, your stress levels will rise. Managing stress and anxiety is an important part of total pregnancy wellness.

Symptoms of Stress and Depression

There are many symptoms of stress and anxiety, including, but not limited to:

- losing interest in the things you used to enjoy
- loss of appetite
- insomnia
- using sleep as a coping mechanism
- lower self-esteem
- a sense of hopelessness / helplessness

- anxiety and/or panic attacks
- breathing issues
- forgetfulness and irritability

If you experience one or more of the above symptoms, talk to your doctor. Your mental state affects your unborn child. If you are experiencing mild problems, mood elevating juices are an excellent supportive strategy. Here's some to keep you going.

KARMA GREEN

2 apples
1 lemon without the peel
1 stalk of celery
1 orange
1 handful spinach

Celery calms the nerves, while the lemon helps to control high blood pressure and reduces mental stress. The pectin in apples also fights bad cholesterol.

SLEEPY TIME JUICE

Juice 2 stalks of celery and 1 lemon in the juicer and add RAW honey to help relax and aid a good night's sleep.

Headaches

Headaches are a recurring problem in pregnancy that can progress to a migraine. Doctors recommend against most over-the-counter remedies.

I believe natural cures and treatments are the safest

option.

Increased blood circulation and hormonal fluctuation are the primary causes of headaches during pregnancy. They can also result from

- dehydration
- low blood pressure
- lack of your usual caffeine fix
- depression and anxiety
- sleep deprivation

Headaches during the first trimester often subside during the second. In the third trimester, you might be suffering the effects of poor posture due to the weight of the baby.

Maintaining good blood sugar levels goes a long way toward fending off headaches.

Fruits that are excellent for this purpose include

- **lime**
- **oranges**
- **pineapple**
- **apples**

To control the amount of fructose you're consuming, mix fruits with vegetables. Better still make sure you eat as much fruit as possible – focusing on juicing vegetables.

CARROT HEAD SMOOTHIE

6 large organic carrots
2 oranges
1 cup (240mls) filtered water
1 apple
1 lime
¼ pineapple

Juice the carrots, oranges and apple. Then add to the blender and add the pineapple lime and water. The oranges in this mixture help to rid the body of toxins, while the complete blend supports good hydration.

THE HYDRATOR

5 carrots
2 cups of spinach
2 apples
1 cucumber
1 cup (240mls) coconut milk
1 grapefruit

An excellent source of Vitamins A, B, C, and K, brilliant for dehydration and thus reducing headaches.

Insomnia

Insomnia is extremely common, before, during and after pregnancy. There are many natural sleep remedies to help this condition that pose no harm to your unborn child. This can be complicated to resolve as there can be many pregnancy related causes for your nocturnal restlessness.

Morning Sickness (at Night...)

More often than not, morning sickness or nausea can plague you during the first trimester. This problem can occur at any hour of the day and even during the night, depriving you of valuable sleep.

Excessive Urination

During pregnancy, especially during the third trimester, the pressure on the bladder increases. Ironic as it may be, drinking water and lots of fluids helps to fix this problem.

Cranberry juice, in particular, is the perfect cure to help remove bacteria encircling the bladder. Blueberry juice has the same effect.

Restless Leg Syndrome

With restless leg syndrome unsettling aches and pains in the legs create a constant urge to move. At night, it can be impossible to get comfortable long enough to get adequate rest.

Natural Insomnia Cures

Juicing and incorporating key herbs offers a natural and healthy cure for insomnia. The herb valerian grows in parts of Europe and Asia. It is a recognized cure for insomnia, thanks to its soothing and calming effect. In a 2008 study, a control group that used valerian for 28 nights fell asleep faster and slept longer than their counterparts.

Consider adding valerian to any soothing, stress relieving juice, or drink a cup of valerian tea at bedtime. Cherry juice has a similar effect for treating insomnia and is also easy to mix into existing juice recipes. (Remember that celery has a calming effect, thanks to its high calcium content.)

Cramping

The internal and external changes during pregnancy can really cause discomfort and irritation. As the baby grows and the uterus expands, the abdominal aches and pains will fluctuate.

This is common and natural, resulting from uterine contractions in response to the baby's growth. Cramping may occur when you sneeze, cough and change sides while sleeping. Gas, indigestion, constipation, and sexual intercourse also cause cramping during pregnancy.

For severe pain with bleeding, seek medical attention. These can be the first signs of premature labour or miscarriage. Cramping may also be a sign of an ectopic pregnancy, where the fetus is growing outside the uterus.

The following juice can be really helpful with cramping

CELERY CRAMPER

**3 ripe tomatoes
1 large handful of spinach
2 handfuls of parsley**

1 pepper
1 cucumber
2 carrots
3 stalks of celery
1 lemon

Urinary Tract Infections

Urinary tract infections are also a frequent cause of abdominal pain. This gorgeous cranberry juice recipe will hopefully offer significant relief.

CRANBERRY RELIEVER

3 fresh oranges
1 Lemon
2 cups (480mls) filtered water
3 cups (375grams) of cranberries
¼ cup agave nectar

Fill a pot with hot water and bring it to a boil. Add the cranberries. Turn down the heat and let it simmer on low heat for about 25 minutes. Remove the mixture from the heat and allow it to cool before blending with the remaining juiced ingredients.

Refrigerate and serve when chilled.

Cranberries have high levels of Vitamin C and antioxidants to fight bacteria in the urinary tract.

Indigestion and Heartburn

Research indicates 8 out of 10 pregnant women will

experience indigestion or heartburn. Both share roughly similar causes during pregnancy.

- Hormonal fluctuations
- Increasing pressure on the stomach
- Dietary changes
- Uterine contractions

For heartburn (and constipation) try the following smoothie recipe

ALOE ACID

2 apples
2 cups (480mls) of filtered water
¼ inch ginger
1 lemon (peeled)
½ cucumber
1 celery
2 tablespoons Aloe Vera pulp

Aloe Vera is a multi-purpose healer. It soothes indigestion, but also offers relief from aching joints. Apples are fantastic for the gallbladder, while cucumber relieves lung, stomach, and chest discomfort. Lemon adds flavour and gives your immune system a boost.

In a variation on this smoothie blend the following:

½ carrot
2 apples
1 orange (peeled)
2 tablespoon of Aloe Vera pulp

2 cups (480mls) filtered water
¼ inch ginger

The addition of carrots gives the juice extra supportive qualities for joint pain.

RAW Apple cider vinegar is also an excellent remedy to help reduce stomach acid – this can be added to any of the fresh juices. If I don't add this to juices, then a drink a tablespoon daily.

Ginger will also help the liver to release digestive juices and enzymes to soothe indigestion.

Coriander/Cilantro also has a soothing effect on both indigestion and heartburn. Try this for a calming super herb reliever.

Try this for a perfect refreshing smoothie

CORIANDER CALM

1 Lime (peeled)
Pinch Himalayan Salt
½ bunch of mint
½ bunch of coriander
2 cups (480mls) filtered water
2 apples
½ cucumber

Overheating

It's not only the hot summer season that can be unbearable when you're pregnant - heat and the effects of constant sweat can cause havoc for your complexion in all seasons.

To deal with these problems, double your intake of filtered water. Nothing does more to bring a glow and radiance to your skin. Green tea is a wonderful herbal solution, rich in antioxidants. If you are experiencing inflammation on your skin, make sure you drink green tea at least twice a day.

Moisturize your face, hands and legs on a regular basis, especially before going to bed at night. Use a good quality scrub to exfoliate your skin at least two or three times a week.

Try using a mixture of yogurt and honey as a natural skin cleanser. Apply the cream to your face for about ten minutes.

The following two recipes are excellent to achieve healthy, glowing skin.

SCRUB 'N' SHINE SMOOTHIE

1 handful parsley
1 handful coriander/ cilantro
1 peeled banana
1 fresh lemon
1 pear
1 apple
3 celery stalks

2 cups (480mls) filtered water
½ lettuce

Blend together with adequate filtered water (this is equally delicious juiced if you prefer....)

SWISS SKIN

2 handfuls Swiss chard
1 inch piece of ginger
1 beetroot
4 carrots
2 oranges

Juice this and your skin will LOVE you forever...

Chapter 7 - Post-Pregnancy Juicing

During the first months of life, breast milk offers great nutrition for your newborn child. However, not all mothers can nurse this way and you should not feel guilty or worry that your baby isn't receiving appropriate nutrition. If you are nursing, make your baby's nutritional needs your top priority when considering your food intake.

While you may be worried about shedding the extra pounds, be aware that your milk is your baby's "all in one" meal. It must contain adequate nutrients to support the infant's growth and development.

Studies reveal that nursing mothers feel even hungrier than they do during pregnancy. An understandable reaction from a system completely engaged in producing breast milk.

Your own nutritional reserves are the "RAW material" the body needs to support lactation. Whatever you eat replenishes those stores. Your body constantly craves more food to create the necessary energy just to keep up!

Managing Your Dietary Intake

On average, a lactating mother requires 500 more calories per day than a woman who is not nursing, which means approximately 2500 calories per day. You should incorporate the usual proteins, fats, grains, fruits, and vegetables in your diet according to very roughly the following levels

- 3 servings of protein
- 5 servings of calcium
- 1 serving of iron
- 2 serving of Vitamin C
- 4 servings of leafy greens
- 8 cups of water, liquids or juice
- 3 servings of whole grains

Even with these rough estimates, you should be able to create a diet plan that will suit your needs. Consider healthy foods like

- Chicken and other lean cuts if you eat meat
- Salmon if you eat fish
- Non GMO organic tofu
- Low fat dairy products if you are able to tolerate dairy
- Brown rice
- Legumes
- Quinoa

While you are working to include these items in your diet, avoid or limit the following

- Alcoholic beverages
- Coffee
- Seafood*

* Although seafood has rich nutritional content, a baby's system is too fragile to handle any mercury that might be present in the fish, especially mackerel and tile fish.

Breastfeeding and Juicing

While you are breastfeeding you will be trying to help your body return to its previous shape in the face of numerous challenges. Food cravings during pregnancy are notorious, however the desire to indulge in forbidden foods or to binge eat can continue during the time you're nursing your child. Add to this the complications of sleep deprivation and an irregular schedule = one disastrous diet......

Juicing and smoothies can be an indispensable aid for curbing cravings. Helping you to take charge of meal timings and will in no way harm you or your baby. In fact, juicing offers numerous benefits for both mother and child:

- **Weight loss** - With minimum solids to digest, the body turns to fat reserves that can be burned to release energy. The act of breastfeeding itself, initiates considerable weight loss in new mothers. With regular juicing, up to 2.5 pounds of weight can be lost in just 2 weeks.

- **Increased energy** - Feeding your child several times a day can be exhausting. When freshly squeezed juices and smoothies are part of your diet, energy levels spike, helping you to feel refreshed throughout the day.

- **Increase in milk production** - Doctors recommended lactating mothers increase fluid consumption to help them produce more milk. Freshly squeezed juice will ensure high nutritional value as well as increased volume.

- **Detoxification** - A well-planned juicing regimen helps to cleanse and purify the system after the physical, hormonal, and even psychological processes of pregnancy.

To juice responsibly while you are breastfeeding

- Maintain a regular schedule.
- Juice ample servings as soon as you feel hungry.
- Use well-washed vegetables – organic if possible.
- Pick out a variety of fruits and vegetables.
- In order to prevent any toxins from entering your child's system, increase your own intake of water throughout the day.

To help you kick start this new regime, here's a high-nutrition beginner's smoothie that will also help with healthy weight loss during the breastfeeding period.

BERRY BLASTER SMOOTHIE

½ cup (120mls) of live yogurt or nut milk
1 handful of blueberries
1 handful blackberries
1 handful strawberries
½ apple
1 banana

Chapter 8 - Juicing Vegetables for Babies

To help the transition into the toddler stage, semi-solid foods are started at roughly six months in addition to milk or formula. Your baby's immune system begins to grow stronger and the bowel is ready to accept more than liquids.

This is where it gets really exciting.....

This is a perfect time to introduce fresh fruits and vegetables while cautiously monitoring digestion to determine which items will be best tolerated.

Vegetables that are suitable for babies include

- Carrots - neither heavy nor gaseous and rich in nutrients.
- Peas - rich in nutrients, with a sweet taste that makes them idea for blending with water or breast milk.
- Steamed and peeled sweet potatoes – high in nutrition with an excellent soft, naturally sweet texture.
- Steamed squash - also blends well and mixes well with watermelon.
- Tomatoes - offer a sweet and tangy taste, but may be too acidic for some children.
- Green beans - highly nutritious and an excellent growth booster.

Juicing is the best way to monitor what goes into your baby's system. If you purchase processed ready-made baby foods, then this can sometimes be a challenge. Store bought food is usually prepared and processed with preservatives and additives such as sugar, often containing unnecessary amounts of carbohydrates and in some many cases even harmful substances like wax.

When your child is ready for their first vegetables, providing homemade juice or smoothie mixtures made from the freshest and healthiest vegetables of the season is an excellent nutritional choice.

Always start with small portions to make sure your baby's digestive system can accept and tolerate the new food.

Key Nutrients

After six months of age breast milk must be supplemented to meet a baby's daily nutritional requirements. The rapid pace of a child's growth during these months demands good nutrition to ensure the correct development of the organs, brain, and immune system.

Babies need five substances during this crucial period that can be easily added to your child's diet with freshly squeezed vegetable juices.

Calcium

Calcium is essential for developing teeth and bones. In the first two years of life calcium also helps to prevent accidental fractures or cartilage damage as the child becomes more physically active.

While your child is still nursing, dilute the vegetable juices you prepare with breast or an alternative milk source. Many people choose nut milk. As your baby's stomach becomes tolerant of a wider variety of produce, both broccoli and tomatoes are also rich in calcium.

Zinc

Zinc boosts the immune system, protecting your child from illnesses caused by viruses and bacteria. It also plays a role in the repair of cells and tissues and is crucial for cognitive development. Both green peas and beans have a large quantity of zinc and can be easily blended into any juice you prepare.

Vitamins A, D, E and K

Vitamin A supports vision and healthy skin. Vitamin D increases calcium absorption and helps with bone growth. Vitamin K is required for blood coagulation in the event of injury, and Vitamin E is a powerful antioxidant that also aids the growth of the nervous system.

With such crucial growth responsibilities, all these vitamins should be encouraged on a daily basis if possible. Common and rich sources of these nutrients include:

- Vitamin A - carrots, broccoli, sweet potato
- Vitamin D - breast milk and fresh orange juice
- Vitamin K - sweet fruits, spinach, Swiss chard, lettuce

- Vitamin E - spinach, asparagus, tomatoes

Iron

Iron is the most important nutrient required for brain development. Those who are born prematurely should be given iron on a regular basis so they can more easily catch up with their growth and development. A lack of iron contributes to deficiencies that can leave a baby with abnormal muscle coordination. Therefore, including Iron in an infant's diet is very important by making use of vegetables like potato, spinach and avocado.

Vitamin B & C

Vitamin C enhances iron absorption and prevents the onset of conditions like scurvy. Vitamin B promotes healthy metabolic activity and increased muscle tone. Leafy greens are the best sources for both of these essential nutrients.

Considerations and Recommendations

You can begin to juice fresh fruits and vegetables for your child from six months of age forward. The nutrients are easily absorbed in this form and free of the additives present in store-bought baby foods. Juicing is perfectly safe for your child, but there are still considerations and recommendations to follow for maximum effectiveness.

Quantity

Be careful not to overwhelm your child's system with

too much juice, especially when your baby has been receiving exclusively breast milk or an alternative. Most experts agree that 4 ounces of juice per day (about 120 ml) is more than enough for a growing baby.

Sweetness

Highly sweetened juices and smoothies are not recommended for babies. Children who are fed sweet foods at such a young age quickly become averse to other flavours and develop a life-long sweet tooth that contributes to weight gain. Excess sugar in the diet also increases the chances of early tooth decay. If you're afraid the juice is too bland or if your child seems to object to the taste, add fruit for natural sweetness.

Concentration

Dilute juices for young babies at a ratio of 1-part juice to 9 parts breast milk or water, which will help your child's body absorb the nutrients more easily.

Packaged or Fresh

Always use fresh vegetables and juices. Bright orange vegetables like squash, for instance, provide Vitamin A to support bone development and a stronger immune system. With packaged vegetables and juices, there is always the risk of feeding your child an unnecessary or unhealthy additive.

Strain the Juices

Always strain juices before giving them to your baby.

When a juice is poorly blended it contains small vegetable particles that can make it thick and "pasty." Straining the juice prevents any risk of choking.

Use One Vegetable at a Time

Start your baby on a single vegetable and wait a day or two to introduce another. This waiting period allows you to judge whether the child is sensitive to the food.

Baby Friendly Recipes

BABY CARROT JUICE

½ carrot
½ apple
1 cup filtered water

Juice the carrot and the apple in a juicer, thinning with water/breast milk/alternative to achieve the desired consistency.

LITTLE GREEN MACHINE

4 leaves of spinach
½ small apple
1 cup (240mls) filtered water

Blend the greens with the milk or water to make a smooth paste. Add the apple a few chunks at a time until the taste is sweet. Dilute with more water as desired.

ABC JUICE

¼ beetroot
1 carrot
¼ lemon

GRACIOUS GRAPES

½ cup (120mls) coconut water
1 carrot
1 handful of grapes
½ watermelon
½ apple

MAMA MANGO

½ mango
½ cup breast milk/alternative/water
¼ banana

You can literally try any combinations, and most recipes can be made into juices, smoothies or a semi-blended meal. Add water depending on the required consistency.

Chapter 9: Dealing with Post-Pregnancy Issues

At the same time that you are enjoying watching your baby grow and develop, you will also be dealing with your own post-pregnancy issues. These include physical and psychological changes. A healthy juicing routine can not only safeguard your child's nutrition in this critical period, it can also help you to recover from the strain pregnancy has placed on your body.

Post-Baby Weight Loss

Shedding post-pregnancy weight can often be a major concern for new mothers. The psychological impact of seeing your body out of shape can be hard to digest.

Planning to lose the pounds requires both patience and planning. Starting any kind of stringent dietary program may actually result in greater weight gain. The stress of managing a baby and trying to lose weight increases binge eating and emotional-based cravings.

Smoothies and Juices can provide you the additional nutrition and energy you need while supporting detoxification and healthy weight loss. When it comes to RAW vegetable juices I generally don't include those calories...

GO TO JUICE

1 apple
2 handfuls of spinach
1 lemon
1 cucumber
½ pineapple
1 inch ginger
2 sticks of celery

THE PARSLEY SOOTHER

3 medium carrots
1 medium beetroot
1-2 stalks of celery
1 handful of parsley
1 lemon, unpeeled
1-2 cloves garlic

Water Retention

Most women will unfortunately, deal with post-pregnancy water retention. This water weight can be alarming as you grapple with swollen legs, ankles, and feet and an overall sense of discomfort.

The medical term for water retention is edema. The extra blood flowing through the circulatory system when pregnant is about 50% more than normal. The strain affects a major vein, the vena cava that carries blood from the lower back to the heart. As the uterus expands, the vena cava becomes less capable of carrying water and blood back to the heart. The water is forced down via the capillaries to the legs, ankles and feet.

Changed hormone levels can complicate this situation, making it difficult for the body to absorb excess water and pass out as waste. With sodium levels in constant fluctuation, the body retains even more water. The problem does start to resolve as soon as the baby arrives, but often not quick enough for comfort.

Within 2-3 days of giving birth you should begin feeling the need to urinate more often and you may find yourself perspiring heavily. These are natural ways for the body to get rid of the collected water, to speed up this process, increase your intake of fresh filtered water and homemade natural juices.

THE GRATEFUL GRAPEFRUIT

1 whole grapefruit
2 carrots
1 Lemon
½ cucumber
½ fennel

THE EXTINGUISHER

2 apples
1 stalk of celery
½ watermelon
1 handful of Kale
4-6 Basil leaves
1 lemon
2 handfuls of spinach

GINGER PLUS

2 handfuls of baby spinach
1 inch ginger
2 cloves garlic
1 handful of basil
1 lemon
3 tomatoes
½ cup (120mls) filtered water

Ginger is a well-known diuretic and should be used at minimum three times per week. (I use it every day...)

Stretch Marks

Stretch marks are one of the most common results of carrying a child. The most frequent locations are the stomach, thighs, buttocks and chest. The stretching and breaking of elastic fibres under the skin cause the marks as the body expands faster than the skin grows. Difficult to avoid and notoriously difficult to remove. However, over time, with the use of natural, rich nourishing creams such as coconut oil and jojoba and by hydrating the skin with healthy juices, the appearance of the marks improve.

ZINC is absolutely essential in both adding to and protecting the elasticity of skin, including skin recovery and overall skin health. These juices include essential sources of natural zinc – great for overall immune health as well as scarring.

THE ELASTIC TOMATO SMOOTHIE

4 tomatoes
1 handful Spinach
1 cup (240mls) filtered water
1 lemon
1 apple
1 handful blackberries or raspberries
¼ ginger

Blend the tomatoes with water and other ingredients until the mixture is as fine as possible. Even after thorough blending, there may be tomato chunks in the mixture, so if you find this a little off-putting then run it through a sieve to separate the chunks from the juice.

HONEYDEW HEAVEN SMOOTHIE

½ honeydew melon
½ pineapple
2 tomatoes
¼ ginger

RED RAW SMOOTHIE

10 strawberries
3 tomatoes
¼ watermelon
¼ beetroot
½ cucumber

Blend the strawberries with the tomato reducing to a fine paste. Juice the remaining ingredients, mix and enjoy.

Dry Skin

Post-pregnancy hormones cause dry skin as estrogen levels drop and water retention begins to resolve. This dryness may be severe enough to cause brown patches that flake and itch. Increasing hydration is the best method to restore skin to a supple, soft condition.

HYDRATING GREEN JUICE

1 apple
¼ of cabbage
2 handfuls fresh baby spinach
1 lemon
1 Lime
1 cucumber
1 celery stalk
1 handful parsley

CUCUMBER MEDLEY

2 cucumbers
2 apples
1 handful of spinach
1 lemon

(You can also apply plain cucumber juice onto your skin to ease the dryness and provide a refreshed and hydrated appearance.)

CARROT & CELERY STICK JUICE

2 carrots
2 celery sticks
1 cucumber
1 apple

VITAMIN SKIN JUICE

2 carrots
2 sticks of celery
1 handful of alfalfa
1 handful of spinach
1 handful of Swiss chard
1 cucumber
1 small beetroot

Fatigue

Many new mothers suffer postpartum fatigue. No matter how much help and support you have, caring for a newborn is exhausting, especially in the days just after delivery.

This enervating tiredness can go on for weeks, creating a need for you to give your body additional support as it attempts to recuperate from the strain of pregnancy. If you are breastfeeding, the recovery can take longer.

Postnatal fatigue has the potential to turn into postnatal depression, characterized by insomnia, a lack of interest in all activities, as sense of disconnection with your child, and a feeling of deep despair.

Healthy juices that provide better energy and promote proper sleep help to fight postnatal fatigue and depression.

KIWI ENERGIZER SMOOTHIE

1 grapefruit
2 kiwis
½ Apple
2 handfuls of spinach
1 handful Swiss chard

BERRY BERRY TIRED SMOOTHIE

2 large handful blueberries
1 handful strawberries
1 handful blackberries
1 cucumber
1 tsp RAW honey

CITRUS & KALE JUICE

2 oranges
1 lemon
1 lime
½ inch ginger
1 large handful of kale
1 apple
½ cucumber

Insomnia

Hormonal imbalances also contribute to sleepless nights for new mothers. Sleeping pills and relaxants are often out of the question for breastfeeding mothers, but juices and smoothies, especially those flavoured with cherry juice - rich in melatonin can be extremely helpful.

CHERRY BOMBASTIC SMOOTHIE

½ pound fresh cherries
½ cucumber
½ honeydew melon
1 lemon (without rind)
¼ cup coconut milk

CHERRY BLASTER

½ pound fresh cherries
2 apples
1 pear
4 carrots
1 handful cilantro/coriander

SPROUTED CAULIFLOWER JUICE

1 handful of beansprouts
1 handful of cauliflower
2 carrots
2 oranges
1 handful of berries (any will do)

Urinary Incontinence

Urinary incontinence describes either the uncontrollable urge to urinate and / or accidental leakage. These incidents may occur while walking fast, getting up too quickly, laughing hard, or sneezing.

During pregnancy, the muscles controlling the uterus, bowel and bladder become stretched. These muscles, collectively called the pelvic floor, are further pulled out of shape by the baby's delivery. As the muscles become weaker, squeezing the muscles at the bottom of the bladder is more difficult, leading to accidents and uncomfortable urgency. Additional complications can arise from hormonal fluctuations and the action of the uterus as it shrinks and begins to return to its original shape and size.

About a third of new mother's experience incontinence issues that do not resolve for 3-6 months. A balanced diet and a good program of exercises will help to speed up this recovery process.

Although healthy juices are helpful in this recovery, care must be taken to avoid overly acidic fruit juices that will actually make the discomfort worse. For this reason, you may need to reduce your intake of citrus juices like oranges, lime, and grapefruit for a while.

BROCCOLI ON THE ROCKS

1 stalk broccoli
4 large carrots
1 apple
½ cucumber

ASPIRATIONAL ASPARAGUS

4 medium asparagus
3 large carrots
2 stalks of celery
½ cucumber

GINGER PARADISE

1 apple
4 carrots
½ inch ginger
1 cucumber

Afterword

Whether you're a juicing fanatic like me, or just keen to improve both your own and the health of those you love - juicing has to be one of the healthiest pursuits possible – the only danger is that of over exhilaration and the pure excitement that comes with controlling the future of your health.

Keep it up, stay focused and you will literally see the changes both physically and mentally in a very short time.

Your body and your baby will thank you.

Afterword

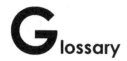Glossary

Acid Reflux Disease: In medical terms, this is referred as 'Gastroesophageal reflux disease' which is a condition during which the acidified liquid contents of your stomach reflux back into the esophagus. Heartburn is known to be the common symptom of this disease.

Acidity: This is a condition in which there will be an excessive amount of gastric juice. This would make the person feel uncomfortable.

Additive: This is a substance which when added in small quantities would enhance, preserve or alter the taste of the product.

Alkaline: A substance will be called as alkaline when it contains alkali (a base) that has the ability to neutralize an acid.

Anemia: This is a medical condition in which there will be a lack of red blood cells in the bloodstream. Anemia will lower the ability of the bloodstream to carry oxygen thereby leading to tiredness, weakness and breathing difficulties in persons who suffer from this condition.

Anticoagulant: This is a substance which would prevent the clotting of blood. These are used for treating the disorders that would show abnormal blood clotting.

Anti-Inflammatory: This term refers to the nature of the substance that could decrease the inflammation (swelling).

Assimilate: This is the act of consuming and incorporating the nutrients into the body. During assimilation, the food will be incorporated into the tissues by the process called anabolism.

Beta-Carotene: This is a pigment that can be found in dark green- and yellow-colored vegetables and fruits. This is known to act as an antioxidant and would protect cells against damage due to oxidation.

Biotin: One of the vitamins in B-complex which is water-soluble in nature. This is important for the enzyme activity. Large quantities of biotin are found in liver and egg yolk.

Bromelain: This is the protein extract from the stems of pineapple. This is a popular culinary agent which is often used as a 'meat tenderizer'. This is actually an enzyme that works to break down protein.

Caffeine: This is a stimulating compound found in coffee, tea, and some other plants. This would taste bitter and is white in color. This is also diuretic.

Calories: This is the unit which is used for measuring the energy that is supplied by the food and released by oxidation. In terms of food, this is otherwise called as kilocalorie or food calorie which is equal to 1000 small calories (gram calories).

Carotenoids: These are the pigments that are seen in the plants and in some bacteria and fungi. These will be red or yellow in color and are structurally similar to carotene.

Cartilage: This is a solid and flexible connective tissue that can be found in various parts of the respiratory tract. This is widespread in the skeleton of newborns and will be replaced by bones during development.

Cellulite: The subcutaneous fat beyond the skin which would look bumpy as it is pushing against the fibrous connective tissues. This often appears on the pelvic region, limbs, and abdomen.

Centrifugal: Centrifugal refers to being operated by using 'centrifugal force' which means moving away from the central axis.

Cervix: This is the cylindrical neck of the tissues that joins the vagina of the women with the uterus. During delivery, this would dilate broadly and allow the baby to pass out.

Chemotherapy: This is a type of cancer treatment that involves the use of chemicals. Most often, the chemotherapeutic agents would be the anti-cancerous drugs and will be administered with a curative intent or reduce the symptoms of cancer.

Cognitive Development: This refers to the development of thought processes like problem-solving, remembering and so on when a child goes to the adolescence and when an adolescent goes to the adult age.

Constipation: This is a condition in which a person would find it hard to evacuate the dry toughened feces from his/her bowels. This could be the result of any functional disorder or intake of improper diet.

Contagious: A disease will be called as contagious when it has the ability from spread from person to person through direct (physical) or indirect (secretions, objects...) contact.

Contaminant: This is a substance when added in sufficient quantity can badly affect the living organisms.

Cramping: This is a sudden involuntary contraction of muscles which will be sometimes accompanied by severe pain. In the lower abdomen, cramping will be experienced by the women during the Day 1 or Day 2 of the menstrual cycle. This will be due to the contraction of the uterus.

Decongestant: This is a pharmaceutical agent that is used in relieving the nasal congestion. This would work by shrinking the swollen membranes of the nose thereby making the breathing process easier.

Dehydration: This is a condition in which there is a lack of water in the body and could result in the breakdown of metabolism. This is caused due to a more amount of water loss compared to the water intake by a person.

Detoxifying: This is the process of removing toxic substances from any living organism. This can be either physiological or medicinal.

Diuretic: This is a substance which elevates the urine production thereby leading to the excretion of water content from the body. In the medicinal field, these are used for treating the conditions like heart failure, water poisoning and so on.

Ecological Balance: This term refers to the state of equilibrium where different organisms coexist with one another and with their surroundings. This represents the stability in the number of each species in the ecosystem.

Elastic fibres: These are the bundles of proteins that are found in the extracellular matrix of the connective tissues. These are rich in the protein – elastin and have elastic property.

Elasticity: This refers to the quality of being elastic.

Ellagic acid: This is a compound that is got from various fruits and has the potential to stop the growth of tumor cells. This will be yellow in color and has the ability to inhibit blood flow.

Essential Nutrients: These are the nutrients that are needed for the physiology to function normally but cannot be synthesized in our body. We should intake these nutrients through our diet.

Estrogen: This is a female sex hormone which is important in the developing and regulating the female reproductive system as well as the sex characters.

Exfoliate: This is the process of removing dead cells from the surface of the skin.

Fatigue: This is a condition of extreme weariness which is usually caused by physical and/or mental exertion. Sometimes, this would also result from illness.

Fetus: This is the unborn human in the womb of the pregnant mother. A fetus is the unborn baby after the embryonic stage (after the 8th week of conception) and before the moment of delivery.

Flavonoids: These are the class of secondary metabolites that are produced in plants. These are believed to give health benefits via cell signaling pathways and antioxidant properties.

Folic Acid: This is one of the vitamins in the B-complex and is water-soluble in nature. This would help the complex carbohydrates in our body to get broken down into simple sugars that could be used for energy.

Folk medicine: This denotes the traditional medicine that usually involves the plant-derived treatments. Examples include Ayurveda, Unani, and Traditional Chinese Medicine.

Gestational Diabetes: This is a medical condition in which a woman who has not been diagnosed with diabetes shows higher blood sugar levels during pregnancy. Most commonly, this would be seen during the third trimester of gestation.

Glycemic Index: This is the value that would indicate the effect of particular food on the blood glucose levels of a person. A glycemic index of 100 is equivalent to the pure form of glucose.

Gout: Gout is a medical condition which is the result of abnormal metabolism of uric acid and would result in the excess amount of uric acid in body tissues and blood stream. This disease has several probable consequences like arthritis, kidney stones and so on.

Heart Arrhythmia: This is a condition of irregularity in the heartbeat. The heartbeat of the person with heart arrhythmia would have their heart beating too fast, too slowly, too early or too irregularly.

Heartburn: This is a condition in which a person would experience burning sensation in the chest. Sometimes, this sensation could extend up to the neck and throat. This is considered to the primary symptom of acid reflux.

Hemoglobin: This is a pigment and protein that is present in the red blood cells. This is responsible for carrying oxygen in the blood and contains iron which gives the pigment a red color.

Hemorrhoids: These, which are commonly known as 'piles' are the blood vessels which are seen in the smooth muscles of the rectum as well as the anus. This is normal in our anatomy but, it could become pathological if they get swollen. The inflamed condition will be called as 'hemorrhoidal disease'.

Herbicides: These are the pesticides that are used for controlling weeds in agriculture. These would specifically target the unwanted plants while leaving the plantation crop undamaged.

Hespiridin: This is a flavonoid got from citrus fruits. Most commonly, this is taken from lemons and oranges and can be crystallized. This is utilised in the treatment of capillary fragility.

Horsepower: This is the standard unit used for measuring the power that is the speed at which the work is being completed. One horsepower is approximately equal to 746 watts.

Hydration: This is the process of supplying water to a person for restoring or maintaining the fluid balance.

In Utero: This is a Latin term meaning 'in the womb' of the pregnant mother. This is generally used to describe the state of an unborn baby (fetus).

Inorganic: Any product is considered to be inorganic if it has not been derived from organic life or from the products of organic life. This is opposite form of organic and does not contain organic matter in it.

Insomnia: A sleep disorder during which the person would have trouble in falling or staying asleep.

Irradiated: To irradiate is to expose an object to radiation. Radiation may be from different sources and most often denotes the 'ionizing radiation' that would be done to serve a specific purpose.

Lactation: This is the process of milk secretion by the mammary glands that would lead to breastfeeding. This would occur after childbirth.

Latex: This is a colorless fluid seen in some plants. This would exude when you cut the plant and would coagulate when exposed to air. The constituents of the latex are proteins, starch, and alkaloids.

Listeria: This is a class of bacteria that has the potential to cause various illnesses. They could even cause fatal infections in a special group of people like elderly people, newborns, pregnant women and those with a weak immune system.

Lycopene: This is the red-colored pigment that is found in several berries and fruits. This is a predominant pigment of tomato. This is found to have antioxidant properties and is known to improve the heart health.

Migraine: This is the condition of severe head ache accompanied by sensory signs like nausea, vomiting, sensitivity to light and so on. The pain that is caused by this can often last for several hours or even for days.

Miscarriage: This is the pregnancy loss due to the death of the fetus before it is delivered by the Mother. Vaginal bleeding with or without pain is the most common symptom of this.

Morning Sickness: This is also called as pregnancy sickness which is characterized by nausea and vomiting. Pregnant women can experience this during the first twelve weeks of gestation.

Multivitamins: A dietary supplement which has a combination of vitamins, minerals, and some other nutritional components. They are available in various forms.

Nausea: This is a sensation of discomfort that can precede vomiting. The discomfort can be felt in the upper stomach. When a person is suffering from nausea, it doesn't mean that he/she will definitely vomit.

Neural Tube congenital disorders: These are the defects found in the following regions during birth: brain, spine, and spinal cord. Spina bifida is a common congenital disorder.

Pediatrician: Pediatrician is a medical professional who deals with pregnancy and childbirth. The major concern of this profession is to care for the health of the women during and sometime after pregnancy.

Omega-3: Polyunsaturated fatty acids of which there are of three types. They are involved in the physiology of humans and are significant to the normal metabolism.

Optimal: This is the most favorable degree of something for getting a result under specific conditions.

Organic Juicing: Juice which doesn't have any chemical or additives. In simple terms, organic juice is the juice in its purest form and is free from synthetic food enhancers.

Oxalates: This is a salt of the oxalic acid that is found in plants and has the ability to form an insoluble salt when combined with calcium. By this process, oxalate would interfere with the calcium absorption in the body.

Parasite: This is a living organism that lives and feeds on another living organism to obtain nourishment. In this kind of relationship, the host organism would not have any benefit from the parasite but most often harmed by it.

Pectin: This is a polysaccharide that is found in the cell wall of the plants. This is commonly used as a gelling agent and as a stabilizer in food processing procedures.

Pesticides: These are the substances that are meant for killing pests and are most commonly used in the crop protection. Pesticides are known to protect the crops from weeds, fungi, and insects.

Phenethylamine: This is an organic compound that is known for stimulant and psychoactive effects. This would function as a neuromodulator and a neurotransmitter in the central nervous system of humans.

Phytonutrients: In simple terms, phytonutrients would mean the nutrients we get from plants. These are the natural compounds that can be found in our plant foods and are found to have beneficial effects in promoting good health.

Placenta: This is a temporary, circular organ that is present in the uterus of the pregnant mother and is the contact point between the mother and fetus. Only through the placenta, the fetus would get the oxygen and nutrients from the pregnant mother. Most typically, the placenta is about seven inches in diameter.

Polyphenols: The class of chemicals that are characterized by several phenol units. Although, these are naturally produced, they are also synthesized artificially at present. These are known to play significant roles in the ecology of plants.

Postnatal: This refers to the time immediately after childbirth.

Postpartum: Same as postnatal.

Pre-eclampsia: This is a type of pregnancy complication that often starts after the 20th week of gestation and is characterized by high blood pressure.

There will be indications of damage to other organs like kidneys. If untreated, this can lead to serious complications for both mother and fetus.

Prenatal: This refers to the term of pregnancy before labour.

Preservatives: These are the chemical substances that are added to food products for preventing the growth of microorganisms that could spoil the particular food. Adding preservatives to the food products would reduce the incidence of food-borne diseases.

Pre-term Labour: Labour will be called as 'pre-term' if it occurs more than 3 weeks before the prescribed due date. If the cervix of the pregnant mother begins to open before reaching 37 weeks of gestation, then the mother is said to be in pre-term labour.

Progesterone: This is a principal female hormone that is secreted by the corpus luteum of the ovary. This would play an important role in preparing the uterus to receive as well as maintain the fertilized egg.

Queasiness: This is the condition in which a person experiences nausea and sickness.

Scurvy: A condition that is caused by the lack of vitamin C. This is usually characterized by the bleeding of gums, fatigue, and spots on the skin. Diet rich in Vitamin-C would be the treatment for this disease.

Spina bifida: This is a type of birth defect in which the backbone and membranes around the spine will not be completely closed. This is commonly seen in the lower back.

Stroke: This indicates the sudden death brain cells that would occur when the blood flow to the brain is stopped. According to the region affected in the brain, this would lead to complications like paralysis, coma, and even death.

Thyroid: This is a small gland that is seen near the voice box and is producing hormones that are helping in the regulation of the various functions of the body. This gland is influencing almost all the metabolic processes in our body through their hormones.

Toxemia: Toxemia of pregnancy is the abnormal condition which will be characterized by hypertension and edema. The other complications of toxemia are fluid retention and protein in the urine.

Toxins: These are molecules or proteins that are poisonous and have the ability to cause disease when come into contact or when absorbed by the tissues. Toxins vary greatly depending on the severity.

Toxoplasma: This is a type of parasite that has the ability to cause 'toxoplasmosis'.

Toxoplasmosis: This is a disease that is caused by toxoplasma gondii kind of parasite. Most often, this disease doesn't have any signs but in some people there will be flu-like symptoms. Newborns would have a higher risk of contracting this infection.

Trimester: Trimester refers to the three-month period in human pregnancy. The whole pregnancy has been divided into three parts and each is called as trimester (first trimester, second trimester and third trimester).

Ulcer: An ulcer is an open sore that can be caused due to a gap in either skin or mucous membrane. This could occur on both internal and external surface of the body and often doesn't heal by itself. In some cases, they will be painful.

Unpalatable: If something is said to be unpalatable, it means that the food is not appealing in terms of taste.

Unpasteurized: This is the antonym of 'pasteurized'. To pasteurize is to expose the food item to a higher temperature for a particular period of time in order to kill the bacteria that could spoil the food. During this process, the flavour of the food will be preserved.

Uric Acid: This is the insoluble compound that is got from the breakdown of nitrogenous compounds that are found in foods and drinks. Mostly, this would dissolve in blood, travel to the kidneys and excrete in urine.

Uterine Contractions: This is a condition in which the uterine muscles will get tightened. During menstruation, this would occur more often throughout the cycle and is referred to as 'endometrial waves' or 'contractile waves'.

Vena Cava: This is the larger vein that would take the deoxygenated blood into our heart. There are two veins in humans: inferior vena cava and superior vena cava.

Index

acidity, 33, 35, 56
air tight container, 49
anxiety, 83, 84, 85, 86
Apples, 18, 27, 39, 48,
50, 66, 70, 72, 73, 74,
78, 92
Apricots, 27, 57
Avocados, 28, 31
bacteria, 23, 26, 40, 48,
49, 89, 91, 102
Bananas, 28, 34, 57, 74
Beet root, 62
Bell peppers, 28
bladder, 36, 88, 89, 116
blood supply, 23
bloodstream, 23, 72
brain development, 103
breastfeeding, 98, 99,
107, 114, 115
calcium, 35, 52, 56, 65,
69, 73, 89, 97, 101, 102
Calcium, 45, 101
Celery, 28, 36, 50, 67, 71,
79, 86, 90, 113
Centrifugal, 24, 25, 59
Cherries, 28
Chia, 53, 55
chloasma, 82
cholesterol, 31, 52, 60,
69, 86
circulation, 76, 77, 78, 86
citrus, 50, 56, 60, 76, 116

consistency, 32, 44, 48,
54, 55, 62, 87, 105
constipation, 34, 40, 72,
73, 74, 75, 76, 90, 91
copper, 52, 66
cramps, 56, 60, 90
cravings, 18, 30, 35, 98,
107
Cucumbers, 28, 37, 50,
62
depression, 53, 83, 84,
86, 114
dermatitis, 78
dry skin, 112
edema, 108
energy, 16, 17, 30, 52,
57, 58, 61, 64, 65, 96,
98, 100, 107, 114
fertility, 60, 62, 84
fetus, 19, 23, 90
Folic acid, 18, 31, 39, 60
freeze juice, 49
fruit, 15, 23, 28, 29, 30,
41, 43, 45, 47, 50, 55,
73, 87, 104, 116
Ginger, 23, 32, 41, 42,
43, 57, 63, 77, 78, 79,
80, 92, 110, 117
Goji-berries, 52
Grapefruits, 28
Grapes, 28, 32, 50, 79,
106
grass juicing, 26

Green beans, 28, 100
headaches, 56, 68, 86, 87, 88
herbicides, 27
herbs, 29, 41, 44, 45, 89
indigestion, 34, 56, 90, 91, 92, 93
insomnia, 56, 85, 89, 114
Insomnia, 88, 89, 115
Iron, 18, 71, 72, 73, 103
juicer, 14, 24, 25, 26, 38, 48, 49, 51, 59, 86, 105, 111
Kiwi fruits, 28
lettuce, 48, 56, 95, 102
Maca, 53, 54, 55
magnesium, 32, 35, 52, 65, 70
Magnesium, 60
manganese, 52, 66
masticating, 24, 25, 49
Mastitis, 80
meal replacement, 19, 23
melasma, 82
migraine, 86
miscarriages, 84
morning sickness, 23, 32, 33, 38, 41, 66, 67, 88
muscle aches, 56
nausea, 23, 33, 41, 43, 56, 63, 66, 67, 68, 69, 88
nutrients, 14, 16, 18, 19, 22, 26, 32, 37, 47, 58,
61, 65, 70, 76, 82, 96, 100, 102, 103, 104
Omega 3, 53, 61
Omega Masticating Juicier, 25
Oranges, 28, 35, 69
organic, 19, 20, 22, 26, 27, 28, 48, 49
Peaches, 27, 74
pesticides, 27, 48, 50
Pineapples, 28, 39
placenta, 18, 64, 70, 73
potassium, 32, 34, 35, 36, 37, 52, 57, 58, 66, 69, 70
pregnancy, 13, 17, 19, 20, 21, 22, 23, 24, 30, 32, 33, 34, 35, 36, 40, 41, 43, 44, 46, 49, 53, 56, 58, 60, 65, 66, 70, 71, 78, 83, 84, 85, 86, 88, 90, 91, 96, 98, 99, 107, 108, 112, 113, 116
protein, 16, 52, 61, 70, 71, 97
RAW, 12, 13, 14, 19, 22, 37, 40, 52, 53, 58, 59, 79, 82, 83, 96
refrigerator, 24
restless leg syndrome, 89
sluggishness, 56
spinach, 15, 18, 31, 32, 38, 39, 48, 56, 65, 69, 71, 73, 75, 80, 81, 86,

87, 90, 102, 103, 105,
107, 109, 110, 112,
113, 114
Spinach, 28, 39, 55, 74,
75, 79, 111
stomach, 41, 47, 63, 67,
68, 91, 92, 102, 110
store bought, 23
store juice, 24, 49
StRAWberries, 27
stress, 23, 84, 85, 86, 89,
107
Stretch marks, 110
sugar, 18, 23, 33, 45, 46,
47, 58, 60, 64, 87, 89,
101, 104
sweet tooth, 28
Tangerines, 28
toxic foods, 22
toxins, 22, 23, 27, 32, 67,
74, 87, 99
triturating, 24
turmeric, 24

urinary problems, 56
uterus, 89, 90, 108, 116
valerian, 89
vegetable, 12, 15, 22,
23, 29, 34, 37, 38, 53,
65, 101, 102, 105
Vitamin A, 18, 22, 35, 37,
58, 65, 80, 102, 104
Vitamin B12, 61
Vitamin D, 102
Vitamin K, 32, 102
water, 27, 30, 31, 32, 34,
37, 42, 44, 51, 53, 55,
57, 62, 67, 74, 75, 77,
82, 83, 87, 88, 91, 94,
95, 97, 99, 100, 104,
105, 106, 108, 109,
110, 111, 112
water retention, 108,
112
zinc, 52, 60, 102, 110
Zinc, 60, 102

Made in the USA
Monee, IL
26 December 2019

19537167R00085